SAQ in
Gynecologic Cancers
(Part I) with Model Answers

SAQ in Gynecologic Cancers
(Part I) with Model Answers

Editor
Professor Farhat Hussain
MBBS FCPS (Obs & Gynae)
Professor and Former Head
Department of Obstetrics and Gynecology
Sir Salimullah Medical College, Mitford Hospital
Dhaka, Bangladesh
fhussain1961@gmail.com

Forewords
TA Chowdhury
Abdul Bayes Bhuiyan

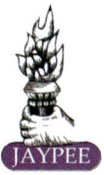

JAYPEE BROTHERS MEDICAL PUBLISHERS
The Health Sciences Publisher
New Delhi | London

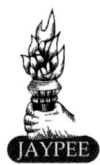
Jaypee Brothers Medical Publishers (P) Ltd

Headquarters

Jaypee Brothers Medical Publishers (P) Ltd
EMCA House, 23/23-B
Ansari Road, Daryaganj
New Delhi 110 002, India
Landline: +91-11-23272143, +91-11-23272703
+91-11-23282021, +91-11-23245672
Email: jaypee@jaypeebrothers.com

Corporate Office

Jaypee Brothers Medical Publishers (P) Ltd
4838/24, Ansari Road, Daryaganj
New Delhi 110 002, India
Phone: +91-11-43574357
Fax: +91-11-43574314
Email: jaypee@jaypeebrothers.com

Overseas Office

JP Medical Ltd
83 Victoria Street, London
SW1H 0HW (UK)
Phone: +44 20 3170 8910
Fax: +44 (0)20 3008 6180
Email: info@jpmedpub.com

Website: www.jaypeebrothers.com
Website: www.jaypeedigital.com

© 2022, Jaypee Brothers Medical Publishers

The views and opinions expressed in this book are solely those of the original contributor(s)/author(s) and do not necessarily represent those of editor(s) or publisher of the book.

All rights reserved. No part of this publication may be reproduced, stored or transmitted in any form or by any means, electronic, mechanical, photocopying, recording or otherwise, without the prior permission in writing of the publishers.

All brand names and product names used in this book are trade names, service marks, trademarks or registered trademarks of their respective owners. The publisher is not associated with any product or vendor mentioned in this book.

Medical knowledge and practice change constantly. This book is designed to provide accurate, authoritative information about the subject matter in question. However, readers are advised to check the most current information available on procedures included and check information from the manufacturer of each product to be administered, to verify the recommended dose, formula, method and duration of administration, adverse effects and contraindications. It is the responsibility of the practitioner to take all appropriate safety precautions. Neither the publisher nor the author(s)/editor(s) assume any liability for any injury and/or damage to persons or property arising from or related to use of material in this book.

This book is sold on the understanding that the publisher is not engaged in providing professional medical services. If such advice or services are required, the services of a competent medical professional should be sought.

Every effort has been made where necessary to contact holders of copyright to obtain permission to reproduce copyright material. If any have been inadvertently overlooked, the publisher will be pleased to make the necessary arrangements at the first opportunity. The **CD/DVD-ROM** (if any) provided in the sealed envelope with this book is complimentary and free of cost. **Not meant for sale.**

Inquiries for bulk sales may be solicited at: jaypee@jaypeebrothers.com

SAQ in Gynecologic Cancers (Part I) with Model Answers

First Edition: **2022**

ISBN: 978-93-5465-645-3

Printed at Nutech Print Services - India

Dedication

*I dedicate this effort to
Women with gynecologic cancer, both living and in our memories,
who has taught us tenacity, selflessness, and courage.*

*My loving parents who raised me with passion for
caring and eternal learning
My husband Professor Zahidul Haq whose enduring support
in academic endeavor provided the strength.*

*My high spirit son, Redwan who is the focus
of all inspiration and
Lastly my brothers and sisters—Shimu, Sohail, and Naz
who are my power in all hardships.*

Dedication

Contributor

Sumaya Akter MBBS FCPS (Obs & Gyne)
Assistant Professor
Popular Medical College and Hospital
Dhaka, Bangladesh
sumaya.akter@yahoo.com

Foreword

It is a matter of great pleasure for me to write a foreword for the book, *SAQ in Gynecologic Cancers (Part I) with Model Answers*, for postgraduate students, edited by Professor Farhat Hussain, retired Professor of Obstetrics and Gynecology who has special interest in the field of gynecological cancers.

This book has been composed in the pattern of Short Answer Questions and their model answers. Though this book does not exempt students from reading standard textbooks on the subject, it will be a good companion for the postgraduate students to do a quick review of the subject. It will also be quite useful to those who are aspiring to take the subspecialty examination in gynecological oncology as it has been compiled in the format of Short Answer Questions, and Bangladesh College of Physicians and Surgeons has introduced this short answer format for fellowship examination of the college.

I hope this book will be well-received by our postgraduate students and prove to be quite useful for a quick revision of the subject.

TA Chowdhury
MBBS FCPS FRCS FRCP FRCOG
Professor
Department of Obstetrics and Gynecology
BIRDEM, General Hospital, Dhaka
President, GOSB, Infertility Society
Past President, OGSB, SAFOG, BMA
Past Chairman, Faculty of Obstetrics and Gynecology
Bangabandhu Sheikh Mujib Medical University Hospital
Dhaka, Bangladesh

Foreword

Foreword

The modern management of gynecological cancer requires a multidisciplinary team approach and benefit to the patients can be given by well orientation of students and junior doctors about this. Significant changes have occurred in the management over the past decade and up-to-date short answer question (SAQ) book in this field is a welcome addition to the wide range of textbooks currently written on the subject.

This book covers seven common gynecological cancers where wide range of knowledge domain which are tested in written assessment has been included starting from basic core knowledge to higher cognitive thinking. It will allow both students and fellow in training to undergo brainstorming and refine their knowledge by practicing and indulging in self-assessment. This book will be a valuable addition to the bookshelves of all aspiring young students and specialists involved in gynecological oncology.

The Editor–Professor, Farhat Hussain, is one of the pioneer in the field of Gynecologic Oncology in Bangladesh. Her passion for the subspecialty is the driving force for this book. She has dedicated most part of her career to the care of women suffering from female cancers in Bangladesh. With the publication of this book, her obvious contribution in this field will be demonstrable—vast clinical experience, surgical expertise, and dedication toward improving cancer care for women.

Abdul Bayes Bhuiyan
MBBS FCPS FICS
Former Head
Department of Obstetrics and Gynecology
Dhaka Medical College
Past President, OGSB, SAFOG
FIGO Awarded on Emergency Obstetric
Care (EmOC)
Program in Bangladesh

Preface

SAQ in Gynecologic Cancers (Part I) with Model Answers is a short question and answer book dealing with different aspects of common gynecologic cancers. It is intended to be a companion to postgraduate medical students who are preparing to appear in Fellowship and Masters in Science Examinations in Gynecologic Oncology and Obstetrics and Gynecology. It is a guide to written examination. The language is simple. Information are concise with adequate facts. Figures in the book are mostly collections from operations and procedures I have conducted, including histopathological image analysis.

Being a teacher for three decades, I have been blessed with the opportunity to guide both undergraduate and postgraduate students. Apart from teaching and mentoring, my dream was to be able do something for students to support their studies. Moreover, being the Head, Department of Obstetrics and Gynecology, Sir Salimullah Medical College, Mitford Hospital for the last 5 years, I was in close association with students of different levels conducting research, pursuing Continuing Medical Education (CME), and working on their thesis or dissertations. I realized students need intensive guidance from their teacher/mentor to do well in an examination. So as part of my vision for a book, I planned to dedicate myself to this project after my retirement. Lastly, the appeal from students for classes, guidance for examination was the final source of motivation and inspiration for writing this book.

In 2020, the Bangladesh College of Physicians and Surgeons (BCPS) brought a change in the written examination where short answer question (SAQ) was introduced. The students were not well oriented with the format and were looking for avenues to solve their problem. They had undue fear regarding the method of assessment because it is based on practical aspects and there are very few books and model questions available. I took the initiative to start the process of writing a book that took nine months from July 2021.

The book is based on my extensive clinical and teaching experience. Besides, input from students who performed well in the written examination as well as those who did not was incorporated in the book. The questions are mostly problem-solving which assess both recall knowledge and its application to higher cognitive thinking. The evaluation and principles of management given in this book are in accordance with the guidelines of International Federation of Gynecology and Obstetrics (FIGO) and National Comprehensive Cancer Network (NCCN). I intended the book to be student friendly and valuable for fellows in training, fellow colleagues, and professionals who deal with gynecological malignant patients. The action plan with explanation to diagnose and treat a problem is outlined clearly in the book. The book includes problems encountered regularly in medical practice and their solutions which textbooks do not always clearly mention. I have tried to refrain from indulging in too many high thoughts to make the text easily understandable to the readers.

This book will not only serve as a question bank, but it will also be a useful source for revision, providing the readers with the fundamental knowledge to sit in the written examination with confidence.

The journey of shaping the book to reality could not have been possible without the enormous contribution and hard work of my colleague, Dr Sumaya Akter, who has brilliantly utilized her computer expertise during drafting and gladfully accepted the long-working hours spent on this book. I am sincerely indebted to her for her contribution.

Professor Farhat Hussain

Acknowledgments

My first debt is to following authors of the standard textbooks who have provided me knowledge and critical thinking in the construction of questions and short answers for the book. The authors along with standard textbooks are:
1. Berek and Hacker's Gynecologic Oncology, 7th edition by Jonathan S Berek and Neville F Hacker.
2. Principles and Practice of Gynecologic Oncology, 6th edition by Richard R Barakat, Andrew Berchuck, Maurie Markman, and Marcus E Randall.
3. Textbook of Gynaecological Oncology, by Ali Ayhan, Nicholas Reed, Murat Gultekin, and Polat Dursun.

I express my sincere gratitude to the publisher M/s Jaypee Brothers Medical Pulishers (P) Ltd, New Delhi, India, who efficiently and effectively oversaw the copyediting of the book. Their medical illustrators have skillfully translated the photography into beautiful illustrative drawings. I am grateful to the publisher for allowing me to use few images from their other published books. This has made my job easier in placement of appropriate images in selected sites. M/s Jaypee Brothers Medical Publishers deserve special acknowledgement for that.

I am thankful to Professor Mohammad Kamal, Former Head, Department of Pathology, Bangabandhu Sheikh Mujib Medical University (BSMMU) Hospital, Dhaka, Bangladesh, for enormous support in providing the cytologic and histopathologic images. Every chapter in the book is enriched by three to four such images. Heartful gratitude to sir for your contribution in spite of your busy schedule. This support was further enhanced by Dr Masud Parvez, Consultant Pathologist, Bangladesh Specialized Hospital who has added few more histopathologic images within a short time. I owe my sincere appreciation to Dr Masud for his wonderful contribution.

I would like to acknowledge the faculty of Radiation and Medical Oncology for sharing pictures related with subject. The faculties are:
1. Professor Qumruzzaman Chowdhury, Ahsania Mission Cancer and General Hospital.
2. Dr Md Arifur Rahman, Associate Consultant, Department of Oncology, Bangladesh Specialized Hospital.
3. Dr Ferdous Ara Begum, Assistant Professor, Department of Medical Oncology, National Institute of Cancer Research and Hospital (NICRH).
4. Md Mezbah Uddin, Medical Physicist, Ahsania Mission Cancer General Hospital.

I wish to thank Dr Afroza Chowdhury, Colposcopist, Bangabandhu Sheikh Mujib Medical University (BSMMU), for making the manuscript rich by adding colposcopic images of preinvasive disease of cervix.

I am grateful to Professor Rokeya Anwar, Professor Shahana Parvin, Dr Dilruba Yesmin, Dr Nasrin Hossain of NICRH, and Professor Jannatul Ferdous of BSMMU, for providing operative and resected specimen images. My sincere appreciation to Dr Sharmin Akhter Rupa, Popular Medical College for providing radiological images.

The manuscript would not have come to reality in the form of book without the constant support and relentless determination of Dr Sumaya Akter. She has shown tireless effort in adding captions to the figures, tables, and flowcharts, cropping the images and placing in appropriate position, writing the abbreviations, correcting the spelling. I remain indebted to her for her such extraordinary work.

lastly in shaping the manuscript into book, I must recognize the contribution of Dr Omar Sohel and M Mohiuddin Mubashshir. Dr Omar Sohel devoted his maximum time in computer typing of different chapters of book. M Mohiuddin Mubashshir contributed in the typing of preliminary part of book.

Contents

1. Cervical Cancer Screening and Abnormal Cervical Cytology 1
2. Cervical Intraepithelial Neoplasia 24
3. Cervical Carcinoma 42
4. Endometrial Carcinoma 69
5. Gestational Trophoblastic Neoplasia 93
6. Epithelial Ovarian Cancer 112
7. Adnexal Mass, Germ Cell, and Sex Cord Ovarian Tumor 141

Abbreviations

AFP	Alpha-fetoprotein
AGC	Atypical glandular cell
AH	Atypical hyperplasia
AIS	Adenocarcinoma in situ
AMH	Anti-Müllerian hormone
AML	Acute myeloid leukemia
ART	Assisted reproductive technique
ASC-H	Atypical squamous cells, cannot rule out high-grade squamous intraepithelial lesion
ASCUS	Atypical squamous cells of undetermined significance
BEP	Bleomycin, etoposide, cisplatin
BOT	Borderline ovarian tumor
BSO	Bilateral salpingo-oophorectomy
CBC	Complete blood count
CBE	Clinical breast examination
CC	Cervical cancer
CCRT	Concurrent chemoradiation therapy
CHM	Complete hydatidiform mole
CIN	Cervical intraepithelial neoplasia
CKC	Cold knife conization
CSF	Cerebrospinal fluid
CT	Computed tomography
D&C	Dilatation and curettage
DM	Diabetes mellitus
DVT	Deep vein thrombosis
EBRT	External beam radiotherapy
EC	Endometrial cancer
ECC	Endocervical curettage
EIN	Endometrial intraepithelial neoplasia
EMACO	Combination of etoposide, methotrexate, actinomycin D, cyclophosphamide, Oncovin/vincristin
EMA-EP	Etoposide, methotrexate, actinomycin D, etoposide, cisplatin
EOC	Epithelial ovarian cancer
EP	Etoposide and cisplatin
ER	Estrogen receptor
EUA	Examination under anesthesia
FST	Fertility sparing treatment

GCT	Germ cell tumor
GIT	Gastrointestinal tract
GTN	Gestational trophoblastic neoplasia
HBOC	Hereditary breast ovarian cancer
HGSC	High-grade serous carcinoma
HNPCC	Hereditary nonpolyposis colorectal cancer
HPL	Human placental lactogen
HPV	Human papillomavirus
HR-HPV	High-risk human papillomavirus
HSIL	High-grade squamous intraepithelial lesion
ICRT	Intracavitary radiotherapy
IDS	Interval debulking surgery
IHC	Immunohistochemistry
IMRT	Intensity modulated radiotherapy
IP	Intraperitoneal
IUD	Intrauterine device
IVU	Intravenous urogram
LAST	Lower anogenital squamous terminology
LBC	Liquid-based cytology
LDH	Lactate dehydrogenase
LEEP	Loop electrosurgical excision procedure
LGSC	Low-grade serous carcinoma
LMWH	Low molecular weight heparin
LN	Lymph node
LNG	Levonorgestrel
LSIL	Low-grade squamous intraepithelial lesion
LVSI	Lymphovascular space invasion
MMR	Mismatched repair
MPA	Medroxyprogesterone acetate
MRI	Magnetic resonance imaging
MSI	Microsatellite instability
MTX	Methotrexate
MTX-FA	Methotrexate-folinic acid
NACT	Neoadjuvant chemotherapy
NPV	Negative predictive value
OAR	Organ at risk
OC	Ovarian cancer
OPD	Outpatient department
OS	Overall survival
OTT	Overall treatment time
PAC	Cisplatin, adriamycin, and cyclophosphamide
PARP	Polyadenosine diphosphate-ribose polymerase
PCR	Polymerase chain reaction

PDS	Primary debulking surgery
PET	Positron emission tomography
PFS	Progression-free survival
PHM	Partial hydatidiform mole
PLAP	Placental alkaline phosphatase
PLND	Pelvic lymph node dissection
PO	Postoperative
PORT	Postoperative radiotherapy
PR	Progesterone receptor
PSM	Positive surgical margin
PSTT	Placental site trophoblastic tumor
PTD	Primary tumor diameter
RH	Radical hysterectomy
RRSO	Risk reducing salpingo-oophorectomy
RT	Radiotherapy
SBE	Self-breast examination
SBT	Serous borderline tumor
SCJ	Squamocolumnar junction
SLN	Sentinel lymph node
SSI	Surgical site infection
STIC	Serous tubal intraperitoneal carcinoma
TAH	Total abdominal hysterectomy
TRUS	Transrectal ultrasonography
TVS	Transvaginal sonography
TZ	Transformation zone
USG	Ultrasonography
VTE	Venous thromboembolism
WHO	World Health Organization

Short Answer Questions

Short answer questions (SAQs) are open-ended questions that require students to frame a coherent, concise response integrating the basics of relevant facts and concepts. SAQs remain the best discriminator between the candidates who perform well in the written examination and those who do not. Among the commonly used tools for assessing cognitive domain of students, SAQ carries greater objectivity and reliability in domains like comprehension, interpretation, recall of knowledge and ability of application. SAQ carries greater objectivity and reliability. Thus, wide range of subject areas can be tested. SAQs are time-tested method of assessment of knowledge in national and international examination.

Reasons for Poor Performance in Examination

Insufficient depth of knowledge is a key factor in poor performance of a candidate in written examination. It is evident that either a candidate appearing in examination may fail to understand the content of case scenario provided or by not correctly interpreting the direction provided in the question. Many candidates include irrelevant information in answering question, which wastes time available, thus fails to perform well because of lack of time to complete the examination.

How SAQs are Used in Assessment?

Short answer questions are intended to be used:
- To assess students recall of knowledge and its application to higher cognitive thinking.
- To assess candidates reasoning skills that lies behind a decision-making process.
- To test both theoretical and practical knowledge of student.
- To evaluate students writing ability.
- As self-assessment aid in training and during revision for examination.

Short answer questions are used both in formative and summative assessment.

How SAQs are Designed in this Book?
- Majority SAQs in this book are designed by setting up a scenario and students are asked to construct response using specific problem-solving strategy.
- The scenario in SAQs are clear, unambiguous, and specific reflecting the type of answer expected. In short, SAQs provide students with a focus (types of thinking and content) to use in their response.

- The number of response expected and marks assigned to each question are indicated so that students can limit their answer appropriately.
- SAQs are the representation of the curriculum highlighted within the trainee logbook.

Short answer questions are student-friendly which allow students to generate more in-depth answer. They are stronger than multiple choice questions (MCQs) and there is no scope of guessing. Lastly, they provide teachers with an open window into students' learning—the real purpose of assessment.

But SAQs are not without *limitations:*
1. The evaluation of SAQs result is time-consuming.
2. They do not encourage long-term retention of knowledge. SAQ mainly assesses the basic knowledge and understanding of a topic, i.e., it assesses the low cognitive levels while long answer questions (LAQs) have the ability to assess higher order cognitive function. Thus, for total assessment of students, framing of questionnaire should include both SAQ and LAQ.

The limitations can be overcome by:
- Evaluating the result by different assessors at the same time
- Constructing questions with clear wording and appropriate language
- Higher cognitive function can also be tested if questions are set taking into consideration the intention.

Short answer questions will test mostly core knowledge but at the same time, the book has enough challenging questions to allow stratification of students and rank them. The explanations in each answer will enrich students' clinical and theoretical knowledge and will teach them an assertive examination technique for answering SAQs.

Thus, I hope this book will enable students to have better understanding about SAQs and get themselves prepared for examination.

CHAPTER 1

Cervical Cancer Screening and Abnormal Cervical Cytology

Question 1

Screening is applicable for cancer cervix and different strategies are effective. All recent guidelines [American Cancer Society (ACS), American Society for Colposcopy and Cervical Pathology (ASCCP), and American College of Obstetricians and Gynecologists (ACOG)] have fixed an age for screening of cancer cervix.

1.1. What age is recommended for screening by majority guideline and why? (1.5)
1.2. Which primary screening strategy is the most effective for cancer cervix? Give reasons for the effectiveness. (0.5 + 1 = 1.5)
1.3. Why screening is possible for cancer cervix? Enlist four important facts which are in favor of screening. (0.5 × 4 = 2)

Answer 1.1

Cancer cervix screening is recommended to start at or above 25 years of age. Cervical cancer is very rare below 25 years. Thus, screening below 25 years will lead to overtreatment. Moreover, abnormal cellular changes evident at younger age often return back to normal spontaneously.

Answer 1.2

Human papillomavirus (HPV) testing alone or cotesting both are effective as screening strategy because there is higher rate of detection of high-grade lesion such as cervical intraepithelial neoplasia 2 (CIN2) and CIN3 by both, in comparison to Papanicolaou (Pap) smear. This is attributable as the sensitivity of HPV testing is 96.4% and cotesting 100% while Pap test has sensitivity of 55% only.

Answer 1.3

Cancer cervix can be screened because of the following facts:
- Uterine cervix is an accessible organ.
- Cervical cancer has long natural history.

2. Cervical Cancer Screening and Abnormal Cervical Cytology

- There is propensity of cells to exfoliate form precancerous lesion.
- Existence of a spectrum of histological change from mild atypia through premalignant lesion to frank malignancy
- Presence of valid and acceptable screening test

Question 2

A 28-year-old recently married lady went to outpatient department (OPD) for consultation in regards to screening for cervical cancer.

2.1. Analyze the eligibility of the lady for screening. (1.5)
2.2. What are the different screening strategies? (1 × 3 = 3)
2.3. How long the lady needs to be screened? (0.5)

Answer 2.1

The lady is eligible for screening because the screening for cancer cervix starts at 25 years according to different guidelines (ACS, ASCCP, and ACOG) because cancer cervix is found mostly in women above 25 years.

Answer 2.2

There are three different screening strategies which are as follows:
1. HPV testing is the preferred method of screening every 5 years.
2. Cotesting with cervical cytology and HPV testing every 5 years is also a preferred recommendation in countries where HPV testing is not Food and Drug Administration (FDA) approved as standalone test.
3. If HPV testing is not available, screening is acceptable by cytology alone every 3 years.

Answer 2.3

The lady needs to be screened up to the age of 65 years provided her previous 10 years reports are normal.

Question 3

A 37-year-old lady did cervical smear **(Fig. 1)** for cytology. She wanted to know the details of the test and went to a cytologist to meet her queries.

3.1. How accurate is Pap smear as screening tool? (2)
3.2. Why is the sensitivity of Pap smear low? (2 + 1 = 3)

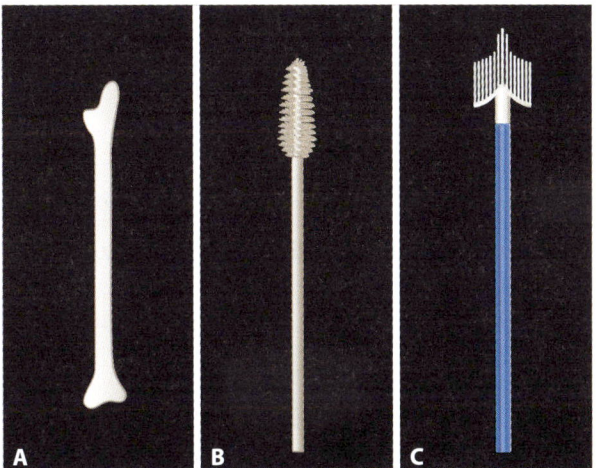

Fig. 1: Sampling device for conventional Pap smear.

Answer 3.1

Pap smear has low sensitivity but high specificity. The sensitivity ranges from 40 to 65% while the specificity ranges from 92 to 96%. Thus, the accuracy in capturing high-grade lesion (CIN2/CIN3) is low.

Answer 3.2

The sensitivity of Pap smear is low because of technical and human error.

Technical errors:
- Failure to capture the entire squamocolumnar junction (SCJ)
- Many cells collected are left behind on the sampling device.
- There is damage and degeneration of some cells on contact with dry slide before fixation.
- Abnormal cells are obscured by blood, mucus, and inflammatory debris.

Human errors: Identification of abnormal cells in Pap smear is dependent on the skill and experience of cytologist.

Question 4

A woman in her late reproductive years went to a cytologist to perform cervical cytology for screening of cervix. She was interested to do cervical cytology which has more diagnostic reliability.

4. Cervical Cancer Screening and Abnormal Cervical Cytology

4.1. Which type of cervical cytology was offered to the woman? (1)

4.2. What information was delivered to explain the difference between recommended cytology and conventional cytology in preparation of Pap smear? (2.5)

4.3. Write three advantages of recommended cytology over other cytology. (0.5 × 3 = 1.5)

Answer 4.1

The cytologist offered the woman liquid-based cytology (LBC) **(Fig. 2)**.

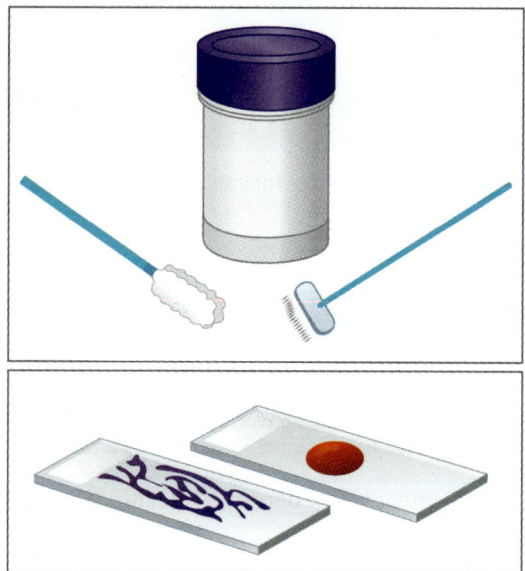

Fig. 2: Liquid-based cytology kit.

Answer 4.2

Liquid-based cytology is different from conventional Pap smear in preservatives and processing machines.

Liquid-based cytology rinses cervical cells in preservatives, processes the solution in machines which separates blood, inflammatory cells, and other obscuring material from epithelial cells.

Thus, homogeneous monolayer smear is prepared on the slide for microscopic evaluation.

Answer 4.3

Liquid-based cytology has improved sensitivity than conventional cytology due to preparation of a thin monolayer smear resulting in:
1. Increased detection rate of abnormal smears
2. Reduction in the rate of unsatisfactory smears
3. Residual cellular material remains available for other tests, e.g., high-risk human papillomavirus (HR-HPV) testing and biomarker tests.

Question 5

A 32-year-old lady received report of conventional cytology which stated enlarged nucleus with increased Nuclear Cytoplasmic ratio (N:C) with varying size and shape. Binucleation is evident with typical koilocytes. The cells are mature which retain polygonal shape with eosinophil cytoplasm.

5.1. What is the diagnosis of Pap smear with the above microscopic feature? (1)

5.2. What are the identification features of koilocytes and what does it signifies? (1.5)

5.3. Outline the action strategy in a flowchart if above cytological report is found. (2.5)

Answer 5.1

The cytologic diagnosis of conventional Pap smear is LS1L **(Fig. 3)**.

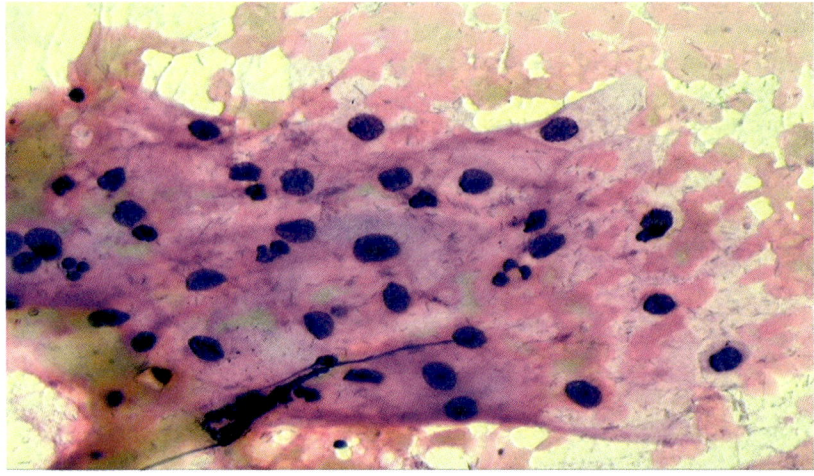

Fig. 3: Low-grade squamous intraepithelial lesion (LSIL) in conventional Pap smear.

Answer 5.2

The identification features of koilocytes are **(Fig. 4)**:
- Well-defined perinuclear halo with eccentric single or binucleated hyperchromatic nuclei
- Dense peripheral rim of cytoplasm

Koilocytes signifies HPV infection and is pathognomonic of LS1L.

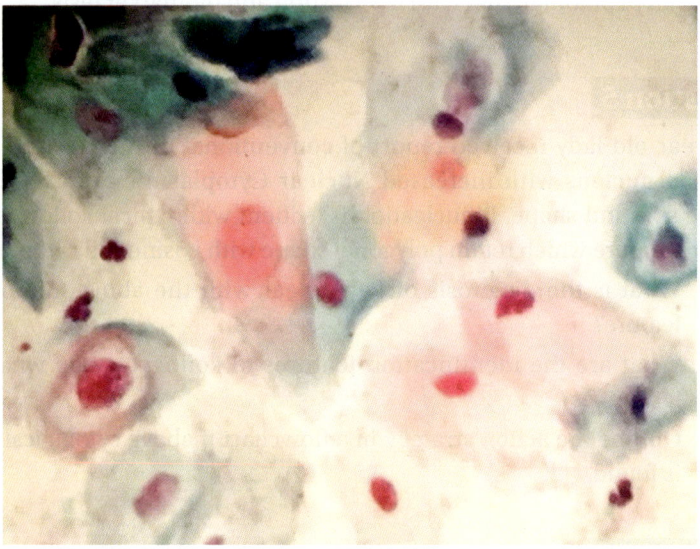

Fig. 4: Features of koilocytes.

Answer 5.3

Action strategy for LSIL **(Flowchart 1)**:

Flowchart 1: Actions in low-grade squamous intraepithelial lesion (LSIL) cytology.

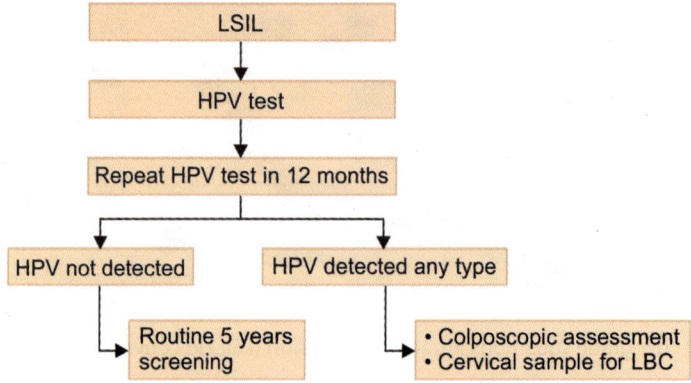

(HPV: human papillomavirus; LBC: liquid-based cytology)

Question 6

A 30-year-old woman did HPV testing **(Fig. 5)** as primary screening test. Since her sister had CIN3, she had queries about HPV testing and went to a cytopathologist.

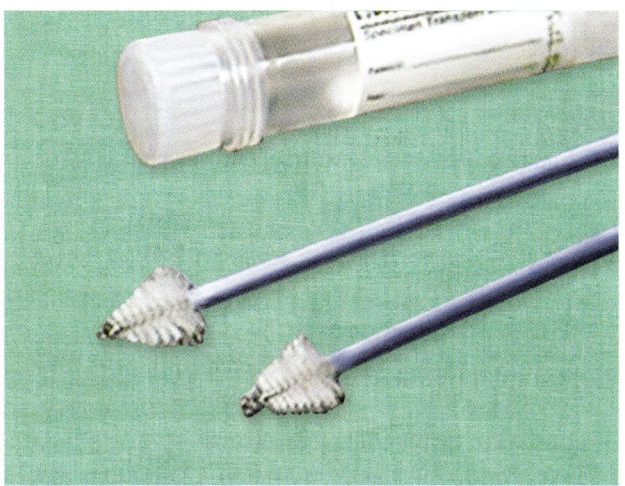

Fig. 5: Human papillomavirus (HPV) testing kit.

6.1. How reliable is HPV testing as a primary screening tool for cancer cervix? (1.5)
6.2. Explain the reason for low specificity of HPV testing in relevance to Pap smear. (1.5)
6.3. Which additional test can identify true precancerous lesion if HPV testing is positive? (2)

Answer 6.1

Human papillomavirus testing is reliable as screening tool because of high sensitivity (96.4%), acceptable specificity (94.1%), and high negative predictive value (100%). Thus, detection of high-grade lesions such as CIN2/CIN3 is high.

Answer 6.2

The low specificity of HPV testing is due to existence of transient infection which is spontaneously eradicated form the body within 12–18 months.

Answer 6.3

Triage test in the form of cytology or partial genotyping are two options that can be used when HPV test is positive to identify disease requiring colposcopy.

- If cytology shows abnormality, referral for colposcopy is done.
- If HPV 16/18 genotyping is done as triage test after HPV positive test, it can identify women with true precancerous lesions. ASCCP now recommends HPV 16/18 genotyping to be performed on women who are positive for HR-HPV.
- If HPV 16 or 18 anyone is positive, the patient should be subjected to colposcopy.

Question 7

Compare HPV testing with conventional Pap test in screening for cancer cervix. (5)

Answer 7

- HPV testing involves detection of HPV DNA in cervical smear while Pap test identifies abnormal ectocervical and endocervical cells.
- HPV test has much higher sensitivity (96.4%) than Pap test (55%) and similar specificity (95% for HPV testing and 97% for Pap test) in detection of high-grade CIN in women between 30 and 65 years of age.
- HPV test is reproducible because machine can accurately and easily identify molecular signs indicating the existence of HPV DNA virus. But Pap test requires skill with experience to identify abnormal cells, thus they are subject to human error.
- HPV testing is done at an interval of 5 years while it is 3 years in Pap test.
- Both HPV test and Pap test have false positivity (30%) and false negativity (10–20%).

Question 8

Persistent HR-HPV infection **(Fig. 6)** is a necessary condition for the development of cervical cancer. But there are variations in HPV types, age group affected and type of HPV infection produced which constitute the natural history of persistent HPV infection.

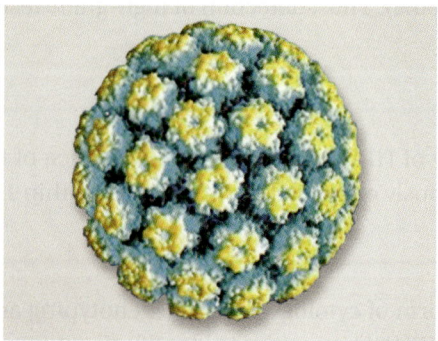

Fig. 6: Human papillomavirus (HPV).

Cervical Cancer Screening and Abnormal Cervical Cytology

8.1. Which 12 HPV types are strongly correlated with cervical cancer? Name the above classified HPV group according to International Agency for Research on Cancer (IARC). (1 + 0.5 = 1.5)

8.2. Which age group of women have high prevalence of HPV infection? What is the characteristic feature of that HPV infection? 0.5 + 1 = 1.5)

8.3. Differentiate two different types of HPV infections produced by HR-HPVs. (2)

Answer 8.1

- HR-HPVs which are strongly correlated with cervical cancer are HPV 16, 18, 31, 33, 35, 39, 45, 51, 52, 56, 58, and 59.
- According to IARC, they are classified as class I carcinogens.

Answer 8.2

- In age group <25 years, HPV infection has highest prevalence. The prevalence rate is as high as 30% in UK, Belgium, and many others countries.
- HPV infection in younger women is asymptomatic and transient. They are spontaneously cleared by host immunity within 12–18 months. Thus, a positive HPV test at this age is misleading and is recommended not to screen women below 25 years by HPV test.

Answer 8.3

Persistent HR-HPV produces either productive or transforming infection.
- Productive lesion is self-limiting that leads to viral shedding causing low-grade lesions—CIN1 and CIN2.
- Transforming lesion progresses to high-grade lesion—CIN2, CIN3, and invasive cancer.

Question 9

A 37-year-old well-to-do-lady wants to do primary screening for cervical cancer. She is eager to select the best screening option and thus seeks assistance from a gynecologist.

9.1. Which test is preferable for her and why? (1.5 + 1.5 = 3)

9.2. Explain—cotesting can also be done as a primary screening test in this woman. (2)

Answer 9.1

- HPV DNA testing is preferable as a primary screening test, because it has increased sensitivity (96.4%), acceptable specificity, and high negative predictive value for detecting high-grade lesion such as CIN2/CIN3 relative to cervical cytology.

- Since the woman is 37 years old, transient HPV infection is less common. 5–10% HPV infection may persist for long time in this age increasing the risk for developing cancer. So, a positive test in such woman carries significance. Again, the woman can afford the test and thus is preferable for her.

Answer 9.2

- Cotesting means performing cytology and HPV testing concurrently. It is done every 5 years in countries where HPV testing is not FDA approved as standalone test.
- Cotesting can also be done in this woman which brings extra advantage, i.e., it increases the sensitivity to 100%.

Question 10

Persistent HR-HPV infection was found in a 35-year-old lady who had primary screening with HPV test and is now on follow-up. She is worried.

10.1. Which viral oncogenes predisposes to the development of HPV associated precancerous lesion? Explain the mechanism by which progression to precancerous lesion takes place. (1 + 2 = 3)

10.2. What are the risk of HPV testing? Explain the consequence of the risk. (1 + 1 = 2)

Answer 10.1

E6 and E7 oncogenes predisposes to the development of HPV-associated precancers lesion.
- After persistent HR-HPV infection, E6 and E7 oncogenes are expressed following integration of HPV DNA with host cell.
- E6 and E7 then degrades/inactivates p53 and pRb, respectively, causing cell survival by impaired apoptosis and cell cycle proliferation. This forms the basis for malignant transformation and progression of disease.

Answer 10.2

Human papillomavirus test carries the risk of false positive and false negative results.
- False positivity may be as high as 30% leading to unnecessary follow-up procedures such as colposcopy and undue anxiety.
- False negativity ranges between 10 and 20% causing delay in appropriate follow-up tests or procedure.

Question 11

Enumerate the role of HPV infection in cervical carcinogenesis. (5)

Answer 11

Human papillomavirus infection and cervical carcinogenesis (Flowchart 2)

- Persistent HR-HPV infection is responsible for 99.7% of cervical cancer.
- Microtrauma disrupts the continuity of cervical stratified epithelium and give access to HPV to the basal layer of squamocolumnar junction.
- In patients with weakened immune system, specific integration of HPV DNA occurs in host cell gene.
- HPV host cell genome then integrates with E2 gene causing increased expression of E6 and E7 oncogenes which inactivate p53 and pRb, respectively.
- Inactivation of p53 ensures cell survival by preventing apoptosis while inactivation of pRb forces infected cells to remain in a proliferative state and escape cell cycle exit.
- The end result of these events is malignant transformation and progression of disease.

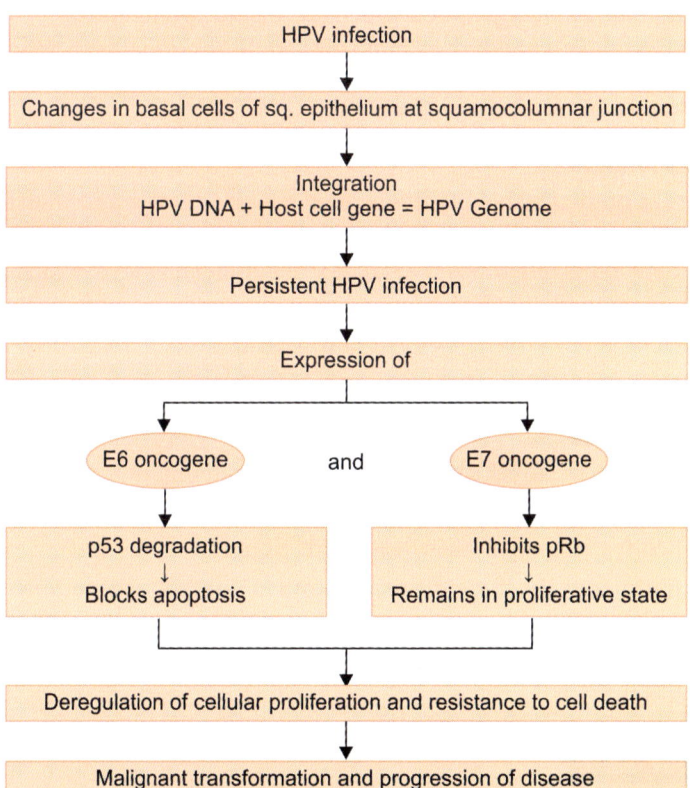

Flowchart 2: Cervical carcinogenesis.

(HPV: human papillomavirus)

Cervical Cancer Screening and Abnormal Cervical Cytology

Question 12

A 42-year-old lady is on regular screening by HPV testing for cervical cancer at 5 years interval.

- 12.1. Compare and justify the difference in the interval between HPV test and Pap test. (1)
- 12.2. If the primary HPV testing is positive, which immediate follow-up option can be adopted? (1.5)
- 12.3. How productive and transforming lesion produced by HR-HPV infection can be detected? (2.5)

Answer 12.1

Human papillomavirus testing is more sensitive and more reproducible than cytology. Thus, safe extension of screening interval can be done at 5 years while Pap test being less sensitive should be screened at an interval of 3 years.

Answer 12.2

The immediate follow-up option which can be advised includes:
- Reflex cytology which can be done to exclude abnormality. If abnormality is detected on cytology, patient is advised for colposcopy.

Answer 12.3

- There is no detectable difference between productive and transforming HPV lesion in cytology or histology at the time of screening.
- The detectable difference is evident at the molecular level which include viral genome integration, reduced viral clearance, and expression of E6 and E7 oncoproteins in transforming lesion.

Question 13

A 33-year-old lady had HPV testing as primary screening which came positive, she attended the OPD for management.

- 13.1. Justify the need of triage test in this woman. (2)
- 13.2. Enumerate the three triage pathways in this lady as recommended by most guidelines. (0.5 × 3 = 1.5)
- 13.3. Which triage pathway will be best in detecting high-grade lesion? (1.5)

Answer 13.1

- Triage test is necessary in this HPV-positive case due to its low specificity.
- It will identify whether she is in need of immediate colposcopy or not.

- Subjecting all HPV positive women to colposcopy will cause increase referrals to colposcopies and overtreatment along with increase in cost which will be beyond acceptable limits.

Answer 13.2

The three triage pathways for above HPV-positive woman as recommended by most guidelines can be any one of the following:
- Cytology
- Dual staining with P16/Ki67
- Partial HPV genotyping for HPV16 and 18

Answer 13.3

Dual staining with P16/Ki67 is the best triage pathway in detection of high-grade lesion. Studies have shown that it has a high sensitivity of 96.6% for CIN3+ among HPV-positive women with normal cytology but positive dual staining.

Question 14

In the current era of HPV-based cervical cancer screening, HPV DNA testing is used as primary screening tool in most developed countries. The details of the test including its impact should be informed to the healthcare providers for their better application in practical field.

14.1. What is the recent impact of such screening on the disease?
$$(1 + 1 = 2)$$
14.2. Enlist the categories of HPV test used in cervical cancer screening.
$$(1 + 1 = 2)$$
14.3. Which methods are commonly used for detection of HR-HPV DNA?
$$(0.5 \times 2 = 1)$$

Answer 14.1

HPV testing has led to a:
- Decrease in cervical cancer incidence and mortality.
- Decrease in proportion of cancer diagnosed at an advanced stage.

Answer 14.2

There are two categories of HPV test that are used:
1. Generic assays test for the presence of 13–14 HR-HPVs as a group and they provide positive/negative results.
2. Partial genotyping assays provide results separately for type 16 and 18 and as a group for high-risk types.

Answer 14.3

- Hybridization with signal amplification
- Genomic amplification using polymerase chain reaction (PCR)

Question 15

A 35-year-old lady underwent HPV DNA test and HPV genotyping, her report was positive for oncogenic HPV 16 and she reported to the gynecologist for management.

15.1. What action should be undertaken now? (1 + 1 = 2)

15.2. If the LBC is LSIL and colposcopy is normal with type 2 transformation zone, demonstrate diagrammatically the actions that should be taken under different situations. (3)

Answer 15.1

- The lady should be subjected to reflex LBC for triaging at first.
- Then she should be referred for colposcopic assessment regardless of LBC result.

Answer 15.2

Actions for LSIL in different situation (Flowchart 3)

Flowchart 3: Diagrammatic representation of low-grade squamous intraepithelial lesion (LSIL).

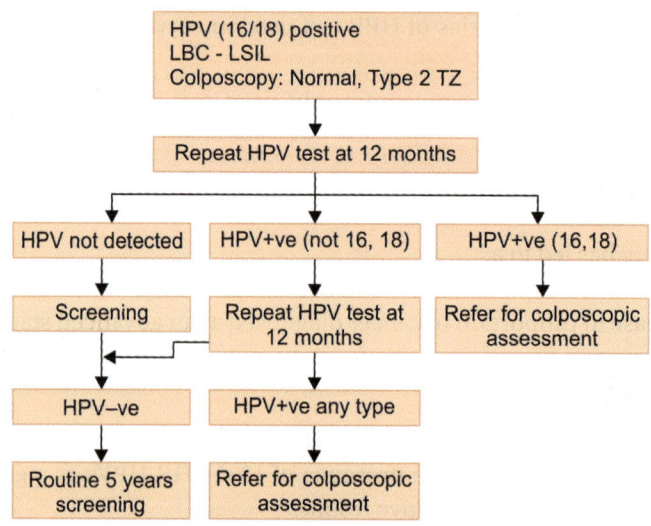

(HPV: human papillomavirus; LBC: liquid-based cytology; LSIL: low-grade squamous intraepithelial lesion; TZ: transformation zone)

Question 16

A 44-year-old lady had conventional cytology as part of regular screening. In the Pap report, there were cells with dark nuclei, irregular nuclear membrane, and high nuclear to cytoplasmic ratios with dense cytoplasm around **(Fig. 7)**.

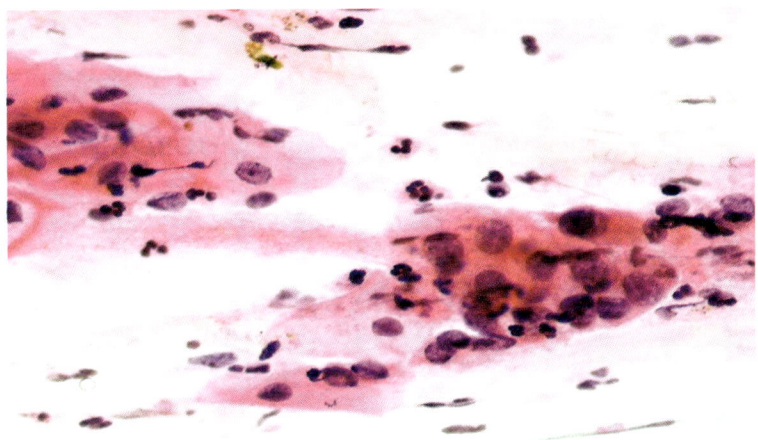

Fig. 7: High-grade squamous intraepithelial lesion (HSIL) in conventional Pap smear.

16.1. What will be the diagnosis of the Pap test? If cytologic features do not fully agree with the above diagnosis, what will be the next diagnosis? (1 + 1 = 2)

16.2. Mention two important conditions that mimics the above diagnosis. (0.5 × 2 = 1)

16.3. Justify the next step of action if above diagnosis is found on Pap test. (2)

Answer 16.1

- The diagnosis will be high-grade squamous intraepithelial lesion (HSIL).
- *Atypical squamous cells:* HSIL cannot be excluded (ASC-H).

Answer 16.2

- Atrophy
- Squamous metaplasia

Answer 16.3

The next step is colposcopy with biopsy because histological specimen will be available for confirmation of diagnosis and exclusion of invasive carcinoma.

16 Cervical Cancer Screening and Abnormal Cervical Cytology

Question 17

A 37-year-old lady with history of postcoital bleeding consulted with a gynecologist. She was advised for LBC and HPV testing. The HPV test was positive for oncologic HPV but not 16/18 and LBC revealed LSIL. She was referred to gynecologic oncologist.

17.1. What is the preferred action? If HPV is detected (not 16/18) again, what step should be taken? (1 + 1 = 2)

17.2. Justify which treatment is preferred if repeat HPV test is positive and LBC report is LSIL. (1.5)

17.3. How frequent is the progression of LSIL into HSIL? Which factor is related to such progression? (1.5)

Answer 17.1

- The patient should have a repeat HPV test at 12 months because HPV test was positive oncogenic type but not 16/18.
- The patient should be referred for colposcopic assessment.

Answer 17.2

Women who have a positive oncogenic HPV (any type) test result with an LBC report of LSIL, who have undergone colposcopy and have a histologically confirmed LSIL, should be kept under observation. She should not be treated because these lesions are considered productive HPV infection which has low neoplastic potential and are spontaneously cleared.

Answer 17.3

The progression of LSIL into HSIL occurs in approximately 9% patients and the risk factor for such progression is HPV 16.

Question 18

A 32-year-old lady had HPV 16 positive in primary screening for cancer cervix. She wanted to have detail information about HPV 16, its risk of persistence, and progression.

18.1. What is risk of viral persistence in this lady? Specify the median time for progression to CIN3. (1 + 0.5 = 1.5)

18.2. What is the role of viral load measurement in this patient? (1.5)

18.3. Enlist four major steps in the development of cervical cancer form HPV 16 infection. (0.5 × 4 = 2)

Answer 18.1

- At 32 years, HPV 16 carries a risk of 8.5% for viral persistence.
- The median time is short, ranging from 5 to 10 years from HPV infection to CIN3.

Answer 18.2

In general, viral load measurement is found to be high in HPV 16 positive infection at enrollment but is of short-term persistence. The course of HPV 16 infection is influenced by many factors such as host immunity, persistence of high viral load, and exposure to established cofactors for HPV progression. Thus, viral load measurement alone plays minimum role for HPV progression.

Answer 18.3

- Infection of metaplastic epithelium of transformation zone (TZ) with HPV 16
- Viral persistence
- Progression of persistently infected epithelium to CIN3
- Invasion

Question 19

A 40-year-old lady received a report stating atypical squamous cells of undetermined significance (ASCUS) in cervical smear. She was called by cytopathologist to explain her current cervical status.

19.1. Explain ASCUS to the lady in simple language along with its clinical significance. (1)

19.2. What are the characteristic features of ASCUS? (2)

19.3. How ASCUS should be managed in this lady? (3)

Answer 19.1

Atypical squamous cells of undetermined significance denotes cellular changes that are more marked than reactive changes but do not meet the criteria for a premalignant disease, i.e., squamous intraepithelial neoplasia.

Clinical significance: Patients with ASCUS for 10–20 years prove to have CIN which are distinctive precursor lesions of squamous cell carcinoma.

Answer 19.2

Characteristic features of ASCUS **(Fig. 8)**:

Nucleus: Single enlarged nucleus, slightly increased N/C ratio, binucleated form with discrete irregularity of nuclear outline.

Cytoplasm: Mature, type of superficial and intermediate or metaplastic cell.

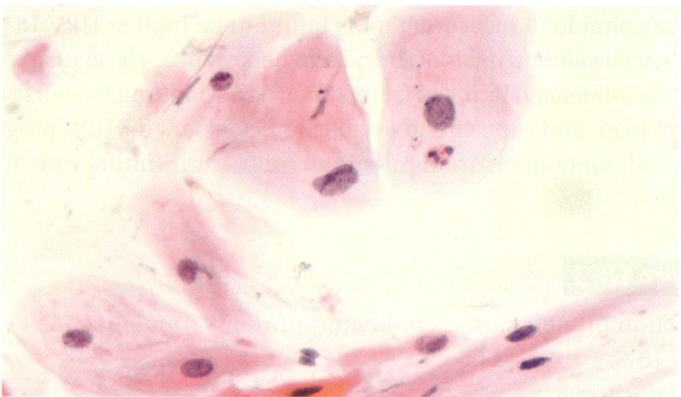

Fig. 8: Atypical squamous cells of undetermined significance (ASCUS) in cervical cytology.

Answer 19.3

According to ASCCP (2019) risk management guidelines, there are three strategic approaches to manage ASCUS.

Flowchart 4: Strategic actions for atypical squamous cells of undetermined significance (ASCUS).

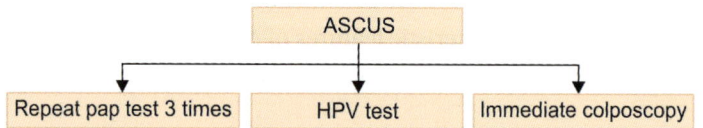

- The above triage tests identify women who have significant disease while sparing others from aggressive and unnecessary procedures.
- HPV triage test is the preferred test because it has NPV of 99.5%.

Since the lady is 40 years, if facilities are available, she should be subjected to HPV test for triaging.

Question 20

A 35-year-old lady reported with excessive vaginal discharge which is occasionally blood stained. Her Pap smear report is HSIL.

22.1. Explain the role of HPV testing for triaging the patient. (1.5)
22.2. Which investigation should be done once HSIL is detected in Pap smear? (1)
22.3. Outline the therapeutic option in relevance to the findings by above investigation. (2.5)

Answer 20.1

90% or more HSIL are associated with HR-HPV. So, there is no role of HPV testing for triaging.

Answer 20.2

Patients should be subjected to colposcopy **(Fig. 9)** and directed biopsy.

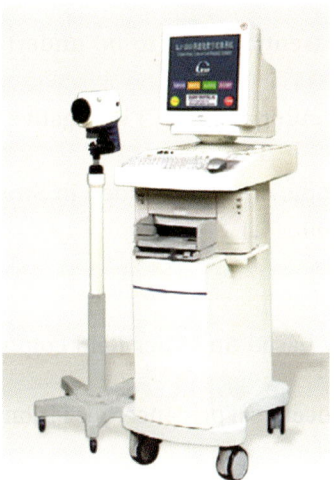

Fig. 9: Video colposcope.

Answer 20.3

- *If colposcopy is satisfactory and biopsy is negative:* Cytology twice at 6 months interval or HPV testing at 12 months is done. If these are negative, the patient resumes her regular screening at 5 years interval.
- *But if colposcopy and directed biopsy shows CIN2/CIN3 or invasive cancer*—treatment will be done accordingly.

Question 21

A 38-year-old lady had colposcopic evaluation of cervix for abnormal Pap test. The colposcopic impression was acetowhite lesion with sharp border but the entire squamocolumnar junction was not visualized **(Fig. 10)**.

Cervical Cancer Screening and Abnormal Cervical Cytology

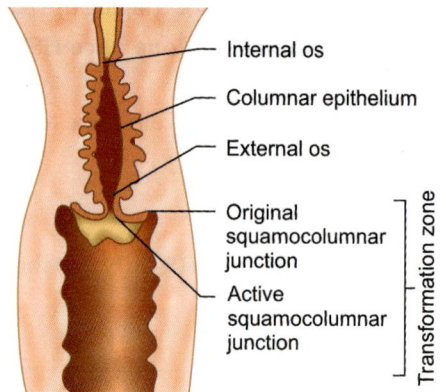

Fig. 10: Transformation zone.

21.1. Mention two essential steps to be undertaken in this situation. (1 × 2 = 2)

21.2. If endocervical curettage (ECC) is negative, what is the next step? (1)

21.3. Which colposcopic criteria is added in Swede colposcopic Index? Justify its addition. (2)

Answer 21.1

- Colposcopic biopsy based on either Reid colposcopic index or Swede colposcopic index
- ECC to exclude endocervical precancerous lesion and cancer

Answer 21.2

The next step is to proceed for excisional cone biopsy.

Answer 21.3

- The lesion size is added in Swede colposcopic index along with other four colposcopic criteria which are present in Reid colposcopic index.
- The implication is that large low-grade lesions may harbor foci of high-grade disease and that size of a low-grade lesion may be a predicator of risk of undetected high-grade disease.

Question 22

An elderly woman who is on regular cervical screening was found to have atypical glandular cell (AGC) in cytology **(Fig. 11)**. She consulted with a gynecologist who advised her for further evaluation.

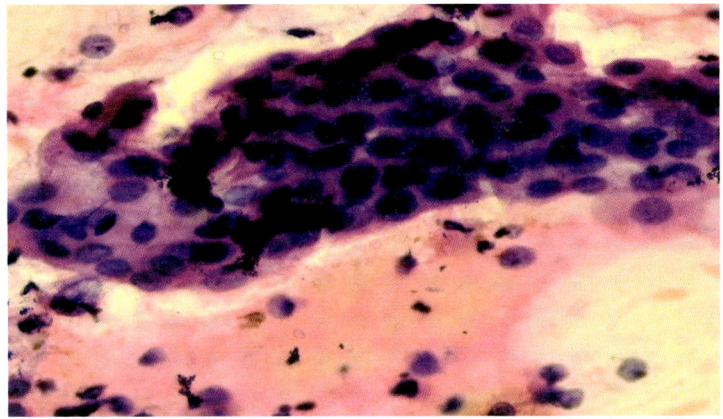

Fig. 11: Atypical glandular cell.

22.1. Why further evaluation is indicated when atypical glandular cell is found in Pap test? (1.5)
22.2. Enumerate the assessment strategy in such situation. (1.5)
22.3. Specify the conditions when special two diagnostic tests are indicated. (2)

Answer 22.1

- Atypical glandular cells in Pap test is clinically significant. It is found in <1% of cervical cytology specimens.
- The risk of premalignant lesion of cervix may be as high as 11%, the risk of endometrial cancer is 3%, while the risk of cervical adenocarcinoma is 1%, which necessitates further evaluation when Pap tests reveal AGC.

Answer 22.2

The assessment strategy includes:
- Colposcopy
- ECC
- Transvaginal sonogram (TVS) to evaluate endometrial thickness, abnormalities in ovaries or fallopian tubes

The above three tests are done in all cases of AGC regardless of HPV result.

Answer 22.3

In following situations, special two diagnostic tests are indicated:
1. If TVS shows thickened endometrium or endometrial polyp, hysteroscopy guided endometrial sampling is done.
2. If colposcopy and ECC are normal, then cone biopsy is indicated to rule out adenocarcinoma in situ or adenocarcinoma of cervix.

Question 23

A 32-year-old lady at 22 weeks of gestation did Pap smear for repeated postcoital bleeding which revealed HSIL, she went to a gynecologist for treatment.

23.1. What immediate action should be undertaken? (1.5)

23.2. If CIN2 is found on biopsy, what will be the treatment plan? (2 + 1.5 = 3.5)

Answer 23.1

Immediate action to be taken is colposcopy with directed biopsy.

Answer 23.2

Treatment plan for CIN2 **(Fig. 12)**:
- Treatment of CIN2 such as ablation or excision is contraindicated in pregnancy.
- If colposcopist is experienced and certain about the absence of invasion based on colposcopy findings alone, the following treatment should be planned:
  - Repeat cytology and colposcopy after 12 weeks, i.e., at 34 weeks of gestation to exclude disease progression.
  - The next colposcopy should be done 6 weeks preferably 12 weeks postpartum when edema, increased vascularity of pregnancy will subside. This will allow less false positivity. If persistent disease is found, specific treatment such as ablation or excision is done.

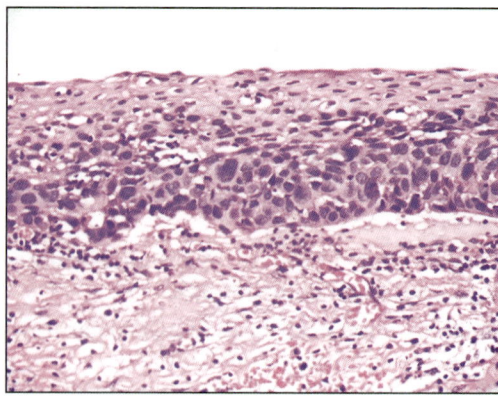

Fig. 12: Cervical intraepithelial neoplasia 2 (CIN2) in histopathology.

Question 24

A 33-year-old lady was referred for colposcopic evaluation following the findings of HSIL in Pap test. There was dense acetowhite epithelium at

6 o'clock position occupying 50% of the lower lip and coarse mosaicism with inner border sign on colposcopic impression. There were also multiple gland openings.

24.1. Which two colposcopy findings are suggestive of severe precancerous lesion? (0.5 + 0.5 = 1)
24.2. What is the role of colposcopic grading system in the evaluation? (2)
24.3. How colposcopic directed biopsy will be collected? (2)

Answer 24.1

*Colposcopic findings suggestive of severe precancerous lesion (**Fig. 13**) are:*
- Dense acetowhite epithelium
- Coarse mosaicism with inner border sign

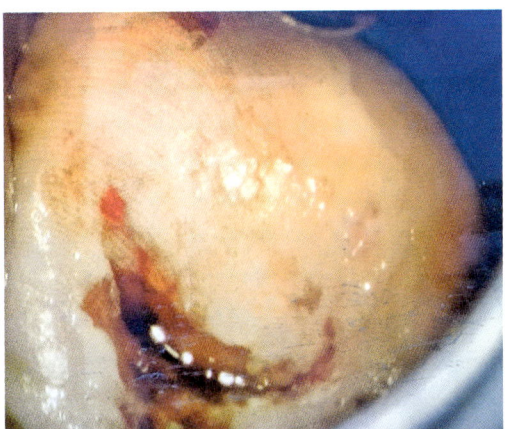

Fig. 13: Colposcopy—severe precancerous lesion.

Answer 24.2

- Colposcopic grading system provides an accurate, reproducible, and clinically meaningful prediction of severity of CIN lesion, enhancing colposcopic-histologic correlation.
- It is not designed to differentiate premalignant from malignant cervical neoplasia.

Answer 24.3

The ASCCP recommendation is to:
- Collect multiple targeted biopsies from areas suggesting severe precancerous lesion, in order to improve disease detection.
- The biopsy should include one form central site of lesion as more severe abnormality is centrally placed according to molecular switch model.

Cervical Intraepithelial Neoplasia

CHAPTER

Question 1

A 33-year-old lady had low-grade squamous intraepithelial lesion (LSIL) on Papanicolaou (Pap) smear. Colposcopy revealed cervical intraepithelial neoplasia 1 (CIN1).

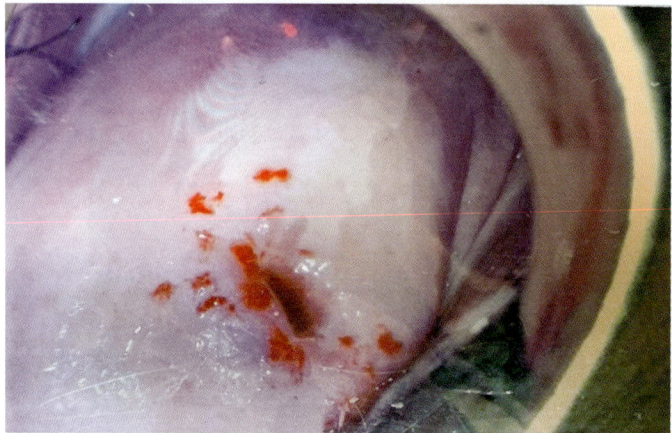

Fig. 1: Cervical intraepithelial neoplasia 1 (CIN1).

1.1. What therapeutic option should be undertaken? Give reasons? $(1 + 0.5 \times 2 = 2)$
1.2. If CIN1 persists after 2 years of follow-up, what should be done? (1)
1.3. Which treatment is preferable in such situations and why? (2)

Answer 1.1

Observation is the preferred therapeutic option because the preceding Pap smear is LSIL, which is a productive human papillomavirus (HPV) infection and undergoes spontaneous regression in most of the time.

Answer 1.2

Immediate treatment in the form of either cryotherapy or loop electrosurgical excision procedure (LEEP) should be done after 2 years of persistent CIN1.

Answer 1.3

Cryotherapy is preferable among the two options as the patient has CIN1 where depth of invasion is minimum (4–5 mm) **(Fig. 1)**. Thus, it can effectively cure the lesion with minimum cost and morbidity.

Question 2

A young 32-year-old lady had colposcopic evaluation of cervix for abnormal Pap smear. The histopathological diagnosis of directed biopsy was CIN2 **(Fig. 2)**. The patient wanted to know the biological behavior and clinical course of disease.

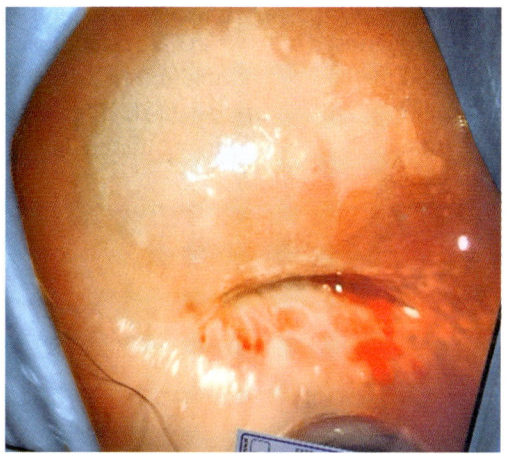

Fig. 2: Cervical intraepithelial neoplasia 2 (CIN2).

2.1. According to lower anogenital squamous terminology standardization project for HPV-associated lesions (LAST)/World Health Organization (WHO), CIN2 belongs to which group of lesion? Is the diagnosis of CIN2 accurate? (1 + 1.5 = 2.5)

2.2. What is the invasive potential of CIN2? (1.5)

2.3. Does the invasive potential of CIN2 remain the same for young patients who are <30 years? (1)

Answer 2.1

- CIN2 and CIN3 are classified together as high-grade squamous intraepithelial lesion (HSIL) according to LAST/WHO.
- CIN2 is a heterogeneous group which is often misclassified. There is high interobserver variability in histological diagnosis with an overall agreement of <50% (i.e., CIN2 are less reproducible). So, the diagnosis of CIN2 is not always accurate.

Answer 2.2

The clinical courses of CIN2 after 2 years shows:
- 50% regression
- 32% persistence
- 18% progression

Answer 2.3

In young patients <30 years, the invasive potential is much lower, i.e., there is higher regression rate and lower persistence and progression rates.

Question 3

A 32-year-old lady was diagnosed as having CIN2 by colposcopy and directed biopsy. She was advised for LEEP to reduce the risk of invasive carcinoma. Her preceding cervical cytology report was LSIL **(Fig. 3)**. But the lady was concerned about her future pregnancy and wanted to defer treatment.

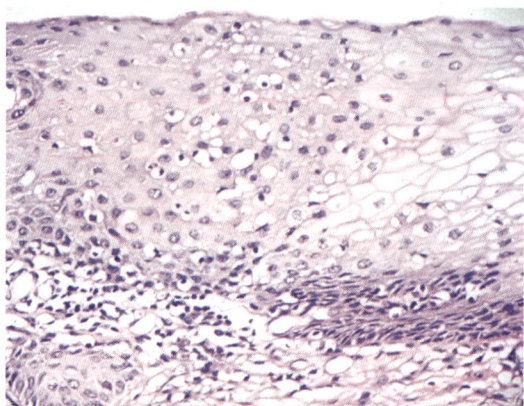

Fig. 3: Low-grade squamous intraepithelial lesion (LSIL) in tissue biopsy.

3.1. How can the lady be helped by the clinician and would it be justified? (2 + 1 = 3)
3.2. How will be the follow-up, if the lady defers treatment? (2)

Answer 3.1

The lady can be kept under observation, because:
- CIN2 is a heterogeneous diagnosis with low reproducibility and high regression rate (30–50%) in young patients. The clinician can allow observation provided:
  - The entire SCJ is visible by colposcope.
  - ECC is negative.

In such situations, the clinician can advise triage test to stratify CIN2 in regards to its invasive potential.

The triage tests are:
- HPV genotyping for 16 and 18
- Immunohistochemistry for P16 or dual staining with P16/Ki67

If these tests are negative, it indicates that the invasive potential of CIN2 is low and it will undergo spontaneous regression in time. Under such circumstances, the lady can be advised to be on observation in a tertiary center under the supervision of an experienced colposcopist.

Answer 3.2

The follow-up during observation will be by:
- *Cytology:* 6-monthly
- HPV testing and colposcopy 12 monthly for 2 years

If two consecutive evaluation shows:
- Cytology < ASC-H
- Colposcopy < CIN2
- HPV result is negative, then:
  - HPV test annually × 3 years
  - HPV test 3 years interval for 25 years

Question 4

A 37-year-old lady underwent a colposcopy for HSIL in Pap smear. The colposcopy and directed biopsy both revealed CIN3 **(Fig. 4)**.

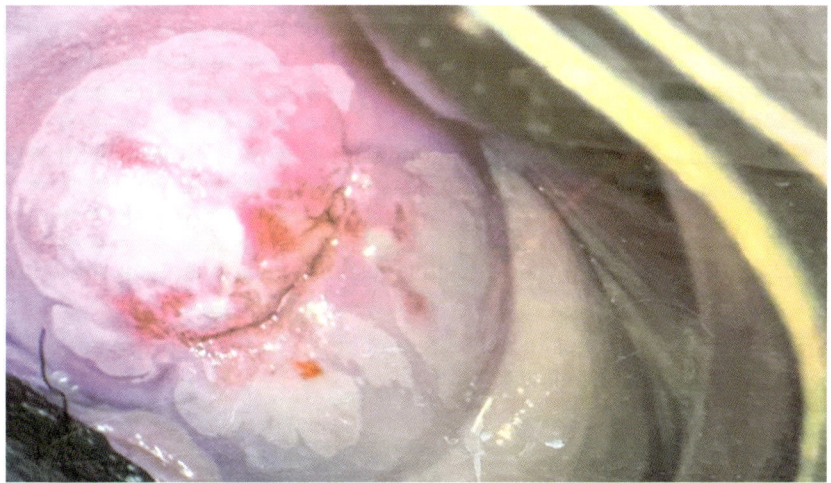

Fig. 4: Cervical intraepithelial neoplasia 3 (CIN3).

4.1. Which treatment option is preferable here? Give three reasons for such preference. (1 + 0.5 × 3 = 2.5)

4.2. Mention the schedule and process of follow-up after treatment. What is the objective of each follow-up in the immediate period? (1 + 1 + 0.5 = 2.5)

Answer 4.1

Excisional treatment in the form of LEEP is preferred.

Reasons for preference:
- The transformation zone (TZ) 8–10 mm is excised including depth of 5–8 mm which allows removing glands of crypts where possibility of abnormal tissue exists.
- Minimum complication occurs following LEEP:
  - Postoperative (PO) bleeding
  - PO infection
  - Cervical stenosis
  - Cervical incompetence
- Allows histological assessment of excised tissue.

Answer 4.2

Patient should be followed up:
- Immediately:
  - After 6 weeks of performing LEEP by history and physical examination to evaluate healing of the wound
  - After 9–12 months by cytology and colposcopy to evaluate regression or persistence of the disease
- Thereafter follow-up should continue for total 25 years.

Question 5

A 35-year-old lady came for consultation with a cytology report of HSIL. She was offered colposcopy which histologically revealed CIN1.

5.1. What will be the next step? (1)

5.2. If the above step yields positive results, which treatment should be offered? (1)

5.3. If the lady wishes to defer treatment, enlist the stepwise approach that should be followed. (3)

Answer 5.1

The next step is to perform HPV testing.

Answer 5.2

If oncogenic HPV (any type) is positive, then patient is offered diagnostic excision of TZ.

Answer 5.3

The stepwise approach during observation should be as follows:
- HPV test and colposcopy at 6–12 months:
  - If both are negative, the woman enters routine 5-yearly screening.
  - If HPV is positive at repeat test, reflex liquid-based cytology (LBC) report is negative or LSIL and colposcopy is normal or LSIL, HPV test should be repeated annually.
  - If HPV is positive at repeat test, LBC is HSIL or any glandular abnormality, she should have a diagnostic excision.

Question 6

A 32-year-old lady had a cervical lesion at 11 and 12 o'clock position of ectocervix (3 × 2) cm in size. The colposcopic evaluation was CIN2 and directed biopsy revealed the same.

6.1. Name the standard treatment in this situation. (1)

6.2. What is the principle of destruction of tissue by the above procedure? (3)

6.3. Enumerate two conditions where high failure rate is found by the above procedure. (0.5 × 2 = 1)

Answer 6.1

The standard treatment in this situation is cryosurgery.

Answer 6.2

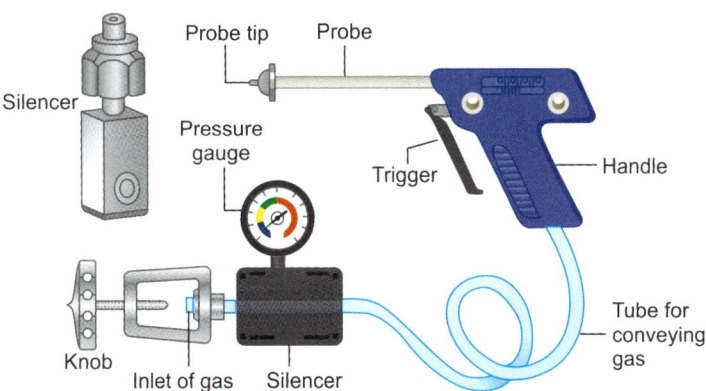

Fig. 5: Cryogun with different accessories.

The principle of destruction of tissue by cryosurgery involves:
- Destruction of tissue, i.e., cell death occurs by crystallization of intracellular water as a consequence of hypothermia produced by evaporation of liquid refrigerants.
- Crystallization begins on the back of cryoprobe and is allowed to continue until the ice ball has extended 7 mm laterally beyond the edge of the probe. This visual landmark indicates 5 mm depth of freezing destroying abnormal tissue.

This process of destruction of tissue involves the use of cryogun with N_2O/CO_2 cylinder **(Fig. 5)**.

Answer 6.3

The two conditions where there is high failure rate are:
1. Large lesion covering the ectocervix.
2. Lesion extending into the endocervical gland.

Question 7

A 32-year-old lady was treated by cryoablation for persistent CIN1 which persisted for 2 years. On follow-up at 12 months, the colposcopy was found unsatisfactory but endocervical curettage (ECC) was negative.

    7.1. What is the recommended treatment? Justify your response.   (2)

    7.2. Enumerate the follow-up procedure. Why follow-up is essential following treatment in this case?   (2 + 1 = 3)

Answer 7.1

The recommended treatment is excisional procedure and the commonly used excisional procedure is LEEP involving insulated Cusco's speculum, wire and ball electrode **(Fig. 6)**, and generator.

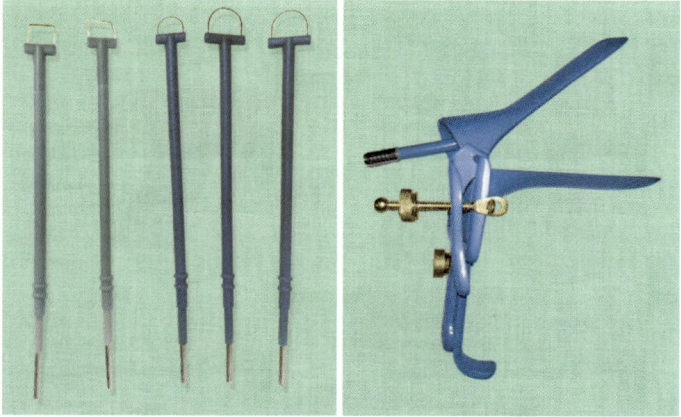

Fig. 6: Loop wire, insulated Cusco's speculum used in loop electrosurgical excision procedure (LEEP).

Loop electrosurgical excision procedure is justified in the above situation because:
- The lesion might be situated within the endocervical canal as the colposcopy is unsatisfactory.
- The woman has been previously treated.

Answer 7.2

The follow-up would be by:
- Physical examination
- HPV test annually or cytology 6 monthly
- Colposcopy annually

When two consecutive results are negative, the woman will return to routine screening at 5 years interval.

Need of post-treatment follow-up:
Post-treatment follow-up is essential in this CIN case in order to detect recurrences early. The treatment failure rate varies between 5 and 15% causing recurrence to happen.

Question 8

A 38-year-old lady with two children was diagnosed colposcopically as having CIN3. She had a big lesion occupying 12 mm area of lower lip of the cervix but colposcopy was satisfactory.

8.1. What is the standard therapeutic option for her? (1)
8.2. How the therapeutic option works to eradicate the lesion? (2)
8.3. How many pass will be needed to excise the cervical lesion? Enumerate the difficulties that will be encountered when such procedure is done. (0.5 + 1.5 = 2)

Answer 8.1

The standard therapeutic option is LEEP.

Answer 8.2

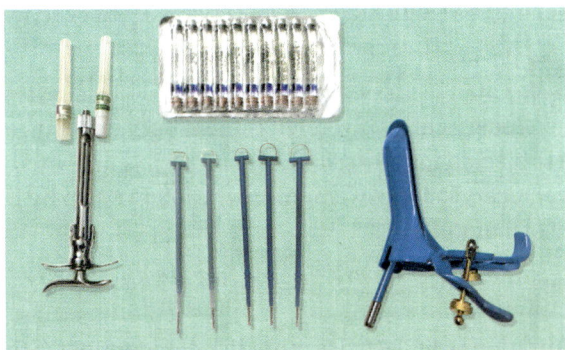

Fig. 7: Instruments on trolley for loop electrosurgical excision procedure (LEEP).

Cervical Intraepithelial Neoplasia

- LEEP cuts off cervix to a depth of 6–10 mm with a low voltage, high frequency radio signal in a tungsten wire **(Fig. 7)**.
- It uses both blended cutting and coagulation, so the area is cauterized as well.

Answer 8.3

- Since the lesion is 12 mm in size, two LEEP passes will be needed to excise the entire lesion.
- The difficulties that will be encountered is in histological assessment which includes:
  - Interpretation of margins
  - Assessment of completeness of excision
  - Evaluation of invasive disease

Question 9

A 36-year-old woman underwent LEEP for CIN3. There was positive surgical margin (PSM) in the histological specimen.

9.1. What is the significance of PSM following LEEP? Outline two important information which are needed for risk factor evaluation. (1 + 0.5 × 2 = 2)

9.2. What will be the approach of management if PSM is present? (1 + 1 = 2)

9.3. Which excision therapeutic modality in CIN carries more risk of recurrence if PSM is positive? (0.5)

Answer 9.1

- PSM after LEEP indicates incomplete excision of CIN3 and is associated with high risk of recurrence and is considered as an independent predictor of recurrence.
- Information which are needed for risk factor evaluation:
  - Size of CIN3 lesion
  - Whether the PSM is included in ectocervical or endocervical component

Answer 9.2

- PSM with endocervical involvement is more risky for recurrence and thus should be subjected to re-excision.
- PSM with ectocervical involvement can be followed up by HPV testing at an interval of 6 months.

Answer 9.3

Cold knife conization (CKC) carries more risk of recurrence if there is PSM.

Question 10

Ablation is one of the therapeutic procedure for CIN. What are the eligibility criteria and disadvantages of ablation? (3 + 2 = 5)

Answer 10

The eligibility criteria of ablation by cryotherapy are:
- Entire lesion should be visible by colposcopy.
- Squamocolumnar junction should be visible.
- The lesion should cover <75% of ectocervix, i.e., cryotips should cover entire lesion.

The disadvantages of ablation are:
- The TZ is not preserved due to freezing. Thus, follow-up by colposcopic evaluation of cervix is unsatisfactory.
- There is delayed healing. It takes 2–3 weeks' time for proper healing of cervix.

Question 11

Compare cryotherapy with LEEP. (5)

Answer 11

- Cryotherapy destroys abnormal cells and surface of TZ by freezing while LEEP cuts and coagulates cervix at the TZ.
- Cryotherapy freezes cervix to a depth of 4–5 mm with liquid N_2O while LEEP cuts and coagulates cervix to a depth of 6–10 mm.
- Cryotherapy is best for smaller lesion, while LEEP is preferred when there is larger lesion or crypt (glandular) involvement.
- Cryotherapy causes less complications than LEEP. There is some risk of cervical stenosis. LEEP causes significant complications such as cervical stenosis and infertility.
- LEEP needs anesthesia while cryotherapy can be performed without anesthesia.
- LEEP provides surgical specimen for histological assessment and evaluation of completeness of procedure which is not available in cryotherapy.
- The follow-up following cryotherapy is difficult because the squamocolumnar junction moves into the os but patient can be followed up easily following LEEP.
- Recurrence after LEEP is lower than cryotherapy in high-grade lesions.

Question 12

A 34-year-old lady underwent LEEP for CIN3. Postoperatively she came to the hospital with problems and communicated with consultant.

12.1. Enumerate five common complications that can occur postoperatively following LEEP. (0.5 × 5 = 2.5)

12.2. How infertility occurs? (0.5 × 2 = 1)

12.3. If patient becomes pregnant subsequently, what is the probable risk? (0.5 × 3 = 1.5)

Answer 12.1

Postoperative complications following LEEP are:
- Burns to the vagina and area of grounding pad
- Postoperative bleeding
- Urinary tract infection
- Cervical stenosis
- Infertility
- Persistent disease at LEEP margin

Answer 12.2

Infertility can occur postoperatively due to:
- Cervical stenosis
- Decreased mucus production form cervical glands

Answer 12.3

The probable risk following conception is cervical incompetence with its consequence like:
- Late spontaneous abortion
- Premature rupture membrane
- Premature delivery

Question 13

A 37-year-old lady who underwent LEEP for CIN3 regularly attended the outpatient department (OPD) for follow-up.

13.1. Why it is important to follow-up the patient following LEEP treatment of CIN3? (1.5)

13.2. Which patients are at increased risk of recurrence following treatment? (0.5 × 3 = 1.5)

13.3. Which test is recommended as "test of cure" following treatment of CIN3? Explain the answer. (2)

Answer 13.1

Women with CIN3 and subsequent treatment with LEEP are at greater risk of residual or recurrent disease. Evidence have shown 4–17% women have CIN2 or greater as a result of residual or recurrent disease following treatment. Thus, follow-up is essential.

Answer 13.2

The risk of residual or recurrent disease following LEEP treatment is associated with:
- Large lesion size before LEEP
- Endocervical extension of the disease
- Incomplete excision of lesion, i.e., PSM of excision specimen

Answer 13.3

- According to recent American Society of Colposcopy and Cervical Pathology (ASCCP) guidelines, woman who have been treated for CIN3 should have cotesting (HPV test and LBC) performed at 12 months and annually thereafter.
- When two negative cotesting are obtained on two consecutive occasions, she can return to routine screening, because the 5-year risks of recurrent high-grade CIN following two negative cotests is minimum (1.5%). Thus the "test of cure" is two negative cotesting.

Question 14

A 32-year-old lady having one child was advised to undergo cryotherapy for CIN2 lesion. She wants detailed information about its use and effect on fertility.

14.1. Which technique should be followed in cryotherapy? Categorize which type of CIN2 can be effectively treated by cryotherapy. (1.5 + 0.5 = 2)
14.2. What is the role of cervical cryotherapy on fertility? (1)
14.3. Comment regarding the use of cryotherapy in pregnancy. (2)

Answer 14.1

- Double freezing technique using a 3-minute freeze, 5-minute thaw, and then 3-minute freeze is the recommended technique of cryotherapy.

- Double-freeze technique is able to extend the ice ball beyond the edge of the cryotip and thus is superior to single-freeze technique.
- CIN2 confined to ectocervix without endocervical extension, with lesion covering <75% area of cervix, so that the cryotip covers the entire lesion are the prerequisite for effective treatment by cryotherapy.

Answer 14.2

Having cryotherapy rarely causes infertility complication. Cervix functions by making watery mucous at ovulation which permits sperm to reach the ovum. This function is not affected by cryotherapy neither there is evidence of cervical stenosis. Thus, fertility is not affected by cryotherapy.

Answer 14.3

- There are limited evidence on adverse pregnancy outcome when cryotherapy is performed during pregnancy; however, an increase risk of pregnancy loss cannot be ruled out. Thus, the recommendation is to defer the patient for cryotherapy during pregnancy and counsel her properly enforcing the need for postpartum visit if CIN lesion is identified during pregnancy.
- Cryotherapy should be performed during postpartum period preferably 3 months after delivery when maximum benefit is gained therapeutically while imparting no harm on the patient.

Question 15

A 42-year-old lady underwent colposcopic assessment for HSIL in Pap smear. The colposcopy was unsatisfactory with nonvisualization of entire squamocolumnar junction.

15.1. What is the next step of action? (1)

15.2. If the next step reveals negative results, explain the strategic plan of treatment. Name the tissues which are removed in the procedure? (1 + 1 = 2)

15.3. Justify which type of procedure will be preferable in this setting. (2)

Answer 15.1

The next step of action is ECC to rule out occult HSIL/CIN3 or invasive cancer within the endocervical canal.

Answer 15.2

- The findings of negative result in ECC with high-grade cytology and unsatisfactory colposcopy as evident in the scenario does not exclude endocervical cancer. Thus, excisional cone biopsy remains mandatory.
- The tissues which are removed by the procedure **(Fig. 8)** include:
  - Ectocervix around cervical os
  - Entire TZ
  - Portion of endocervical canal

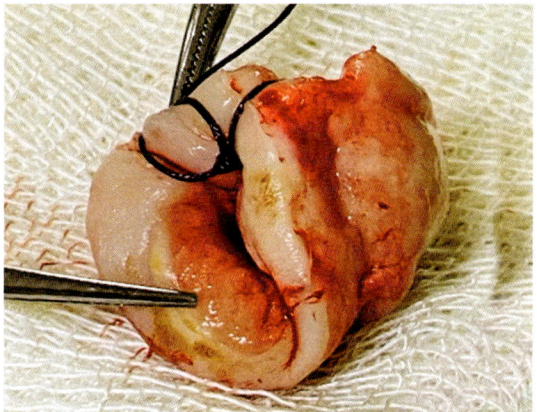

Fig. 8: Cervical tissue after conization.

Answer 15.3

Cold knife conization will be preferable because there will be availability of single surgical specimen without "burned" edges, thus allowing complete evaluation of margins to declare the completeness of treatment. In short, cold knife conization will serve both diagnostic and therapeutic purpose.

Question 16

A 44-year-old lady underwent cold knife conization for significant discrepancy between cytology and colposcopy. In the postoperative period, she had complications for which she needed frequent follow-up.

16.1. Enumerate the two grave complications that was encountered.
(0.5 × 2 = 1)

16.2. Compare the risk of above complications in different conizations.
(1)

16.3. Enumerate the precautions that can be taken to avoid complications.
(3)

Answer 16.1

Two grave complications are:
1. Intraoperative and postoperative bleeding.
2. Cervical infection.

Answer 16.2

The risk of complication is almost same with cold knife, laser, and LEEP conization.

Answer 16.3

Peroperative precaution that should be taken to avoid complication are:
- Bilateral ligation of descending cervical artery before conization to minimize peroperative blood loss.
- Hemostasis by ball electrode of diathermy to prevent oozing from operative bed postoperatively.
- Excision of <1.5 cm of cone to avoid cervical incompetence.
- Dilatation of external os after conization to avoid cervical stenosis.

Question 17

A 37-year-old lady was diagnosed colposcopically as having CIN3 and extension of 1 cm within the endocervical canal and advised for excision. She has completed her family and seeks management.

    17.1. Justify the standard treatment for this lady. (2)
    17.2. What is the role of hysterectomy? (1)
    17.3. How will you follow-up the patient if she needs hysterectomy? (2)

Answer 17.1

The standard treatment in this case should be cold knife conization because:
- It will serve both diagnostic and therapeutic purpose.
- The cure rate will be high with the removal of endocervical component.
- Since the family is complete, the risk of cervical stenosis and cervical incompetence will be manageable.

Answer 17.2

Hysterectomy is not indicated as primary treatment of CIN3. If the lady has coexisting other gynecological condition that warrants hysterectomy, then only it can be done.

Answer 17.3

If the lady needs hysterectomy, the follow-up will be by:
- Vault smear and colposcopy on two occasions within 18 months after surgery.
- Thereafter vault smear and HPV test (cotest) annually, until the lady has tested negative by both tests on two consecutive occasions.

Question 18

A 32-year-old lady had a positive HPV test and cytologic test revealing HSIL. She is now running 12 weeks of pregnancy and wants advice regarding the issue.

18.1. What should be the next step? (1)

18.2. When should colposcopic assessment be done in this lady? Justify your answer. (1 + 1.5 = 2.5)

18.3. Justify if CIN3 is found on colposcopic assessment when should be she treated. (1.5)

Answer 18.1

The next step is to perform colposcopy.

Answer 18.2

- Pregnant woman who meets the criteria of colposcopy can safely undergo colposcopy at 12 weeks and a second assessment in late second trimester. The primary aim of colposcopy here is to exclude invasive disease and to defer biopsy until she has delivered. Evidence has shown that delaying treatment in pregnancy does not have an adverse effect on the prognosis, rather disease persistence at the same stage is found.
- If colposcopy-directed biopsy is deferred until child birth, repeat colposcopy and biopsy is done 3 months following delivery, when edema, abnormal cellular changes, and increased vascularity are reduced, thus interpretation difficulties are overcome.

Answer 18.3

Cervical intraepithelial neoplasia 3 disease needs definitive treatment in the form of LEEP or cone biopsy. This treatment in this lady is deferred during pregnancy because of the risk of excessive hemorrhage and is done safely 3 months following delivery.

Question 19

A 40-year-old lady was diagnosed with adenocarcinoma in situ (AIS) of the cervix. She came to the hospital for better understanding of the disease and management.

Cervical Intraepithelial Neoplasia

19.1. Which type of lesion is AIS? Specify the recommended treatment for such abnormality. (0.5 + 1 = 1.5)

19.2. Justify the recommended treatment mentioning three important points. (0.5 × 3 = 1.5)

19.3. Can completeness of surgery be assured, if conization with clear margins is obtained in young woman wishing fertility? (2)

Answer 19.1

- It is a preinvasive glandular lesion of the cervix.
- The recommended treatment is hysterectomy.

Answer 19.2

- AIS frequently extends for a considerable distance into the endocervical canal making excision difficult.
- AIS is frequently multifocal and has skip lesions. Thus, total removal is essential.
- If conservative surgery such as LEEP or CKC is done and negative margin is obtained, it does not necessarily mean that the lesion has been completely excised.

Thus, hysterectomy is justifiable in such cases.

Answer 19.3

This cannot be assured in AIS because even negative margins in conization carries <10% risk of persistent AIS and small risk of cancer.

Question 20

A 36-year-old lady was diagnosed with AIS of cervix by ECC. Patient opted to conserve the uterus for fertility reason and consulted gynecological oncologist for management.

20.1. What type of conservative management option can be offered to the lady? (1)

20.2. Which parameter must be ensured in the procedure to obtain best outcome? (1)

20.3. Which three important issues the lady needs to be counseled before conservative treatment? (1 × 3 = 3)

Answer 20.1

Excision procedure either CKC or conization by laser therapy can be offered to her.

Answer 20.2

The surgical margins of the excision procedure should be negative of tumor.

Answer 20.3

The lady should be counseled regarding the following issues:
- There is potential risk of residual disease and recurrence even if the surgical margins are negative as fertility sparing treatment is not the standard of care.
- Long-term surveillance annually by cytology and HPV testing must be ensured.
- Definitive treatment in the form of hysterectomy is needed once childbearing is complete.

Cervical Carcinoma

CHAPTER 3

Question 1

A woman with cervical cancer (CC) stage IB1 with cervical growth 1.5 × 1.5 cm **(Fig. 1)** was admitted in the hospital for surgical management. The patient had squamous cell carcinoma, grade 2 in cervical biopsy.

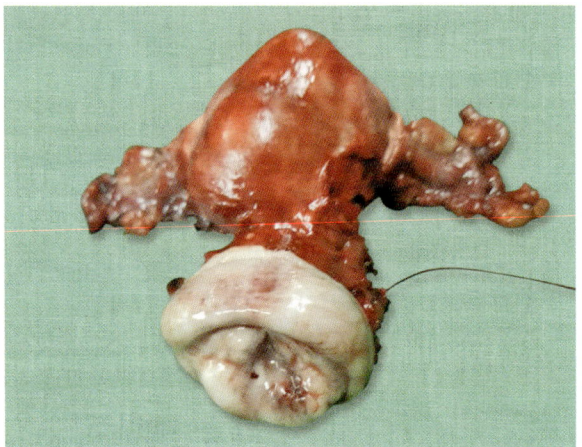

Fig. 1: Resected uterus with cervical growth.

1.1. Which surgical management is appropriate for the patient? (1)
1.2. Justify the role of pelvic lymphadenectomy here. (0.5 × 4 = 2)
1.3. Is laparoscopic-assisted procedure feasible in this case? What are the advantages? (1 + 0.25 × 4 = 2)

Answer 1.1

Radical hysterectomy, type III with pelvic lymphadenectomy.

Answer 1.2

In stage IB1 CC, approximately >15% have positive lymph nodes. So systematic pelvic lymphadenectomy in such cases is helpful to:
- Accurately stage the disease
- Provide therapeutic benefit by resecting bulky positive lymph node

- Stratify patient for adjuvant treatment
- Provide prognostic information

Answer 1.3

Laparoscopic radical hysterectomy with pelvic lymphadenectomy is feasible as the tumor is small in sizes (1.5 × 1.5 cm).

Advantages:
- Less morbidity
- Few blood transfusions due to decreases in blood loss
- Faster recovery
- Shorter hospital stays

Question 2

A 46-year-old lady was diagnosed as stage IIA1 CC, histology subtype—squamous cell carcinoma. She was offered to choose any modality of treatment—surgery or radiotherapy assuring her that both have similar outcomes and efficacy. The patient was convinced to select surgery as the primary treatment.

2.1. Enlist the advantages of surgical treatment. (0.5 × 4 = 2)
2.2. Name the surgery that will be offered to the patient. Specify the sites of division of cardinal and uterosacral ligament. (1 + 0.5 × 2 = 2)
2.3. Outline the extent of pelvic lymph nodes removal. (0.25 × 4 = 1)

Answer 2.1

The surgical treatment provides advantages as follows:
- Accurate staging of disease is possible based on histopathologic findings.
- Individualization of adjuvant treatment.
- Preservation of ovarian function.
- Psychological relief of patient as the disease organ is removed.

Answer 2.2

- Type III radical hysterectomy with pelvic lymphadenectomy
- In type III radical hysterectomy, the division of ligaments is as follows:
  - Cardinal ligament is divided at the pelvic side wall.
  - Uterosacral ligament is divided near sacral attachment.

Answer 2.3

Pelvic lymph nodes which are removed include:
- Parametrial nodes
- Obturator nodes

- External iliac nodes
- Internal iliac nodes
- Common iliac nodes

Question 3

A 43-year-old woman presented with postcoital and intermenstrual bleeding for the last 8 months. On clinical evaluation, there was a barrel-shaped cervix with free fornices and parametrium. Cervical biopsy and endocervical curettage (ECC) revealed adenocarcinoma of cervix, grade 2.

 3.1. What is the preferred treatment in this case? Justify.   (1 + 2 = 3)
 3.3. Mention the schedule of post-treatment surveillance of this patient.   (0.5 × 4 = 2)

Answer 3.1

- The preferred treatment is radical hysterectomy **(Fig. 2)** with pelvic lymphadenectomy.
- In adenocarcinoma histologic type of cancer cervix, radiotherapy is discouraged as primary treatment because adenocarcinoma is generally regarded as radio-resistant in comparison to squamous cell carcinoma. Because of the above concept, as the patient is in early stage, surgery is selected as preferred treatment.

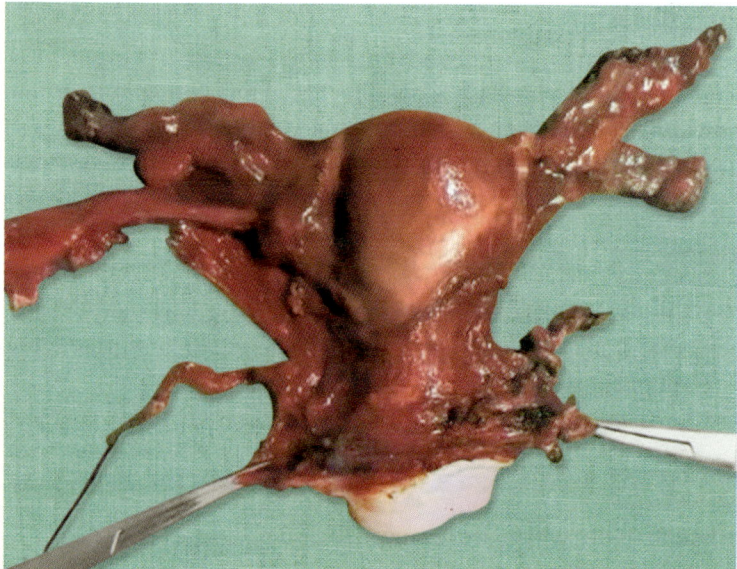

Fig. 2: Radical hysterectomy specimen depicting endocervical adenocarcinoma.

- Moreover, since the patient is young, sexual function can be well maintained following surgery by:
  - Conserving the ovaries
  - Excising shorter length (1.5 cm) of vagina

Answer 3.2

Patient is monitored after treatment to detect early recurrence. The schedule of follow-up is:
- Monthly for first 3 months
- 3 monthly for the next 2 years
- 6 monthly for the next 5 years
- Annually for the rest of life

Question 4

A 42-year-old multiparous lady is diagnosed as invasive CC—squamous cell type, FIGO stage 1B2. She got admitted for treatment.

4.1. What will be the primary treatment for her? (2)

4.2. Mention four important points to differentiate modified radical hysterectomy from radical hysterectomy. (0.75 × 4 = 3)

Answer 4.1

- Either surgery or radiotherapy anyone can be chosen as primary treatment as both have similar outcomes.
- Because of the advantages in young patient, surgery will be preferred.

Type III radical hysterectomy with pelvic lymphadenectomy will be the choice of surgery.

Answer 4.2

TABLE 1: Differentiation between type II and type III radical hysterectomy.

Points	Type II radical hysterectomy	Type III radical hysterectomy
Indication	• Stage 1A1 with LVSI • Stage 1A2	Stage IB1, IB2, IIA
Uterine artery	Ligated just medial to the point at which it crosses the ureter	Ligated at its origin where it branches off the hypogastric artery
Vagina removed	1–2 cm of upper vagina is removed	2–3 cm of upper vagina is removed
Cardinal ligament (Fig. 3)	Divided at the medial half	Divided at pelvic side wall
Uterosacral ligament (Fig. 3)	Medial half is removed	Divided near sacral attachment

(LVSI: lymphovascular space invasion)

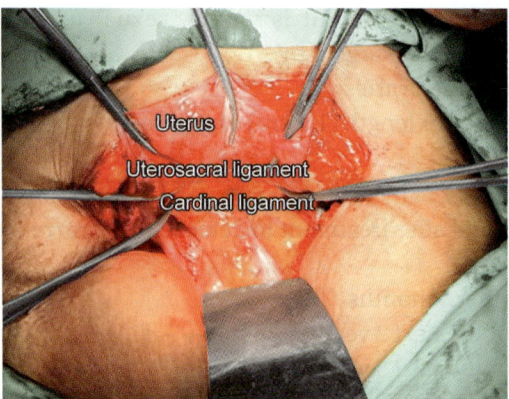

Fig. 3: Division of uterosacral and cardinal ligaments in type II, type III radical hysterectomy.

Question 5

A patient was diagnosed as cervical carcinoma, squamous cell subtype, grade 2. Clinical evaluation revealed a cauliflower tumor (3 × 4.5) cm in the anterior lip of cervix but the fornices and both parametrium were free. Magnetic resonance imaging (MRI) of abdomen showed pelvic lymph nodes enlarged with unilateral hydronephrosis.

  5.1. What is the stage of the disease? Specify the probable reason for unilateral hydronephrosis in this case. (0.5 + 1 = 1.5)

  5.2. What is the standard treatment here? (1.5)

  5.3. If the patient has bilateral hydronephrosis, what treatment should be given? (2)

Answer 5.1

- Stage IIIC1
- The ureter is probably compressed externally by enlarged pelvic lymph nodes causing unilateral hydronephrosis **(Fig. 4)**.

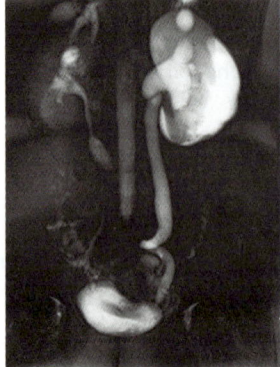

Fig. 4: Magnetic resonance imaging (MRI) urogram showing hydroureter and hydronephrosis.

Answer 5.2

The standard treatment is concurrent chemoradiation (CCRT) but before radiotherapy, resection of bulky lymph nodes via extraperitoneal approach if done will significantly improve the survival of the patient.

Answer 5.3

Renal status should be assessed by creatinine clearance.

If creatinine clearance is <50 mL/min, bilateral ureteric stenting should be done followed by chemoradiation.

Question 6

A 40-year-old woman underwent simple hysterectomy for abnormal uterine bleeding. Invasive CC was found during pathologic evaluation of specimen of uterus.

6.1. How should the woman be evaluated now? (1 + 1 = 2)
6.2. Mention the treatment options for such patient. (1 + 1 = 2)
6.3. If repeat surgery is done, what are the challenges faced by the surgeon? (1)

Answer 6.1

For evaluation:
- The extent of disease should be assessed by:
  - Positron emission tomography (PET)/computed tomography (CT) scan if available
  - If not available, then chest X-ray
  - CT or MRI scan of pelvis and abdomen
- Hysterectomy specimen should be assessed for high-risk features:
  - Positive surgical margins
  - Deep infiltrating tumor
  - Lymphovascular space invasion (LVSI)

Answer 6.2

The treatment option is CCRT provided:
- No evidence of metastatic disease is found
- No high-risk features in hysterectomy specimens

If any of the above is found, the treatment option is repeat laparotomy followed by:
- Radical parametrectomy
- Upper vaginectomy
- Pelvic lymphadenectomy with or without adjuvant CCRT.

Answer 6.3

Repeat surgery is difficult due to previous scarring, adhesions, and distortion of anatomy.

It must be done in centers where experienced surgeons are available.

Question 7

A woman who is clinically diagnosed as early staged CC was subjected to imaging for accurate staging.

7.1. Which imaging is preferable for determining accurate staging of cancer cervix? Give reasons. (1)
7.2. Enlist five information obtained from the imaging tool for accurate staging. (0.5 × 5 = 2.5)
7.3. When PET scan use is indicated? (1 + 0.5 = 1.5)

Answer 7.1

Magnetic resonance imaging having high soft-tissue resolution is the preferred imaging tool to accurately determine the staging.

Answer 7.2

Information that are obtained from MRI include:
- Primary tumor diameter
- Extension to parametrium
- Extension to vagina
- Status of lymph nodes
- Depth of cervical stromal invasion

Thus, accurate preoperative staging can be determined.

Answer 7.3

Positron emission tomography scan has the ability to determine more accurately the extent of disease, particularly status of lymph nodes when they are not enlarged.

Distant site metastasis can be detected by PET scan when they are undetectable by conventional imaging.

Thus, if available and affordable, PET inclusion preoperatively will more accurately assign staging.

Question 8

A woman who was diagnosed as stage IB3 cervical carcinoma with histology of squamous cell carcinoma grade II, reported to hospital for management.

8.1. Which treatment option is most preferred and why? (0.75 × 2 = 1.5)
8.2. What extra benefit is gained by such treatment? (1.5)
8.3. Which imaging is used for treatment planning? What are the other imaging methods which will provide accurate information on local tumor extent? (1 + 0.5 × 2 = 2)

Answer 8.1

Primary chemoradiation therapy is the preferred treatment option.

The reason behind it is as follows:
- When the tumor is bulky like stage 1B3, there is increased probability of lymph node metastasis and early recurrence. This consequence is prevented by giving radiotherapy following surgery. Thus, dual treatment increases morbidity like lymph edema, radiation proctitis, cystitis, colitis, and sexual dysfunction and is discouraged.

Answer 8.2

Since chemotherapy is added with radiotherapy, there is significant improvement in local control of the disease and overall survival (OS) when chemotherapy is added with radiation because chemotherapy acts as a sensitizer of radiation, thereby increasing its efficacy.

Answer 8.3

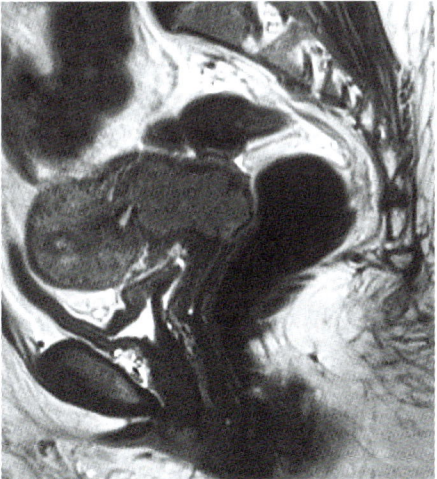

Fig. 5: Magnetic resonance imaging (MRI) showing bulky tumor.

- Magnetic resonance imaging in bulky tumors **(Fig. 5)** like stage IB3 is used in treatment planning.

- The other imaging methods which provide accurate information on local tumor extent in CC are:
  - Transvaginal ultrasound (TVS)
  - Transrectal ultrasound (TRUS)

Question 9

A 56-year-old woman was diagnosed as cervical carcinoma. On clinical evaluation and MRI, she was staged as IIA2.

9.1. Enlist four high-risk factors which are likely to be present in such a stage. (0.5 × 4 = 2)

9.2. Which modality of treatment is preferred here? Give reasons for such preference. (1 + 1 = 2)

9.3. Why is CCRT more favorable than radiotherapy alone in the treatment of cancer cervix? (1)

Answer 9.1

Since the tumor is bulky in stage IIA2, the likelihood of high-risk factors are:
- Positive pelvic lymph nodes
- Positive parametrium
- Invasion of more than half of cervical stroma
- LVSI

The presence of such high-risk factors increases the risk of recurrence.

Answer 9.2

Concurrent chemoradiation is preferred here.

Reasons of preference:
It avoids the severe morbidity associated with dual modality of treatment, i.e., surgery followed by adjuvant radiotherapy.

Answer 9.3

Chemotherapy sensitizes the tissue to the effect of radiotherapy, thereby increasing the efficacy. As a result, patient getting CCRT shows improved OS, progression free survival (PFS), and decreased local and distant recurrences.

Question 10

A 37-year-old married woman with recent history of (H/O) kidney transplantation and on immunosuppressive medications reports with heavy menstrual bleeding. She also complains of bleeding in between menstruation for the last 4 months. She is worried about CC and wants to have a checkup.

10.1. Mention four important other symptoms you want to obtain from her which will suggest cancer cervix. (0.5 × 4 = 2)

10.2. Which examination and investigations suggest parametrial involvement in such cancer? (0.5 × 2 = 1)

10.3. Name four investigations recommended by International Federation of Gynaecology and Obstetrics (FIGO) to be included with clinical examination to assign the stage of disease. (0.5 × 4 = 2)

Answer 10.1

1. Vaginal discharge which may be foul smelling
2. Postcoital bleeding
3. Pain in lumbosacral or gluteal region
4. Pervaginal bleeding on straining

Answer 10.2

- Rectovaginal examination **(Fig. 6)**
- *Imaging studies:*
  - High-resolution ultrasonography (USG)
  - MRI/CT scan

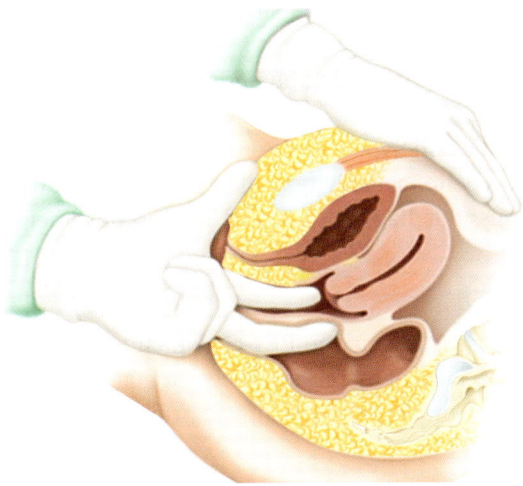

Fig. 6: Rectovaginal examination.

Answer 10.3

- Cervical biopsy
- Chest X-ray

- *Imaging:* USG/intravenous urogram (IVU)/CT/MRI/PET
- If relevant symptoms are present, cystoscopy and proctoscopy.

Question 11

Lymph node status should be meticulously assessed preoperatively in patients with CC.

11.1. Why is reliable information on lymph node status necessary once diagnosis of cancer cervix is confirmed? (0.5 × 3 = 1.5)

11.2. Compare the different imaging tools in the assessment of metastatic lymph node. (2.5)

11.3. How PET-CT assesses lymph node status? (1)

Answer 11.1

Lymph node status is an independent predictor of prognosis, thus preoperatively reliable information about it must be known to:
- Accurately determine staging
- Plan treatment
- Predict the prognosis of disease

Answer 11.2

- Both MRI and CT have low sensitivity in detecting metastatic lymph node. The reasons are:
  - Nonbulky metastatic lymph node may remain unrecognized.
  - Bulky lymph nodes are detected but differentiations between metastatic and hyperplastic enlarged lymph node are not possible.
- PET-CT has better sensitivity in diagnosing metastatic bulky lymph node but may miss the diagnosis in small/microscopic metastasis.

Answer 11.3

F18-deoxyglucose is injected in PET-CT which is taken up by tumor cells in lymph nodes because of increased glucose metabolism.

This results in increased tracer uptake which is then detected by PET-CT.

Question 12

A woman underwent radical hysterectomy with pelvic lymphadenectomy for cancer cervix stage IB1. She was counseled about the procedure.

12.1. Outline the boundary within which pelvic lymphadenectomy should be performed to ensure its completeness. (2)

Cervical Carcinoma

12.2. If 1 cm of external iliac vein is injured during surgery, what will be the principle of repair? (2)

12.3. Which postoperative treatment should be ensured prophylactically to prevent deep vein thrombosis (DVT) following repair? (1)

Answer 12.1

The boundaries for pelvic lymphadenectomy **(Fig. 7)** are:
- *Cranially:* Bifurcation of common iliac artery
- *Caudally:* Deep circumflex iliac vein
- *Inferiorly:* Obturator nerve
- *Medially:* Obliterated umbilical artery
- *Laterally:* Genitofemoral nerve

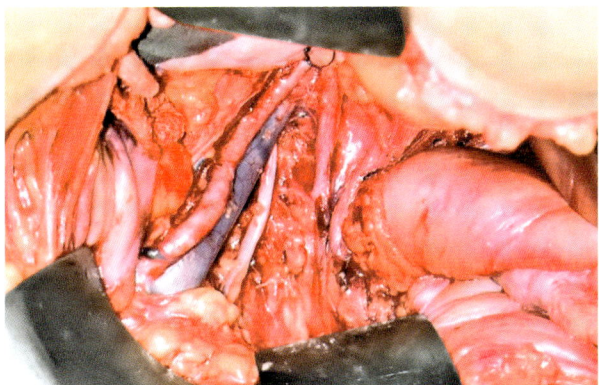

Fig. 7: Boundaries of pelvic lymph node dissection.

Answer 12.2
Principal of Repair

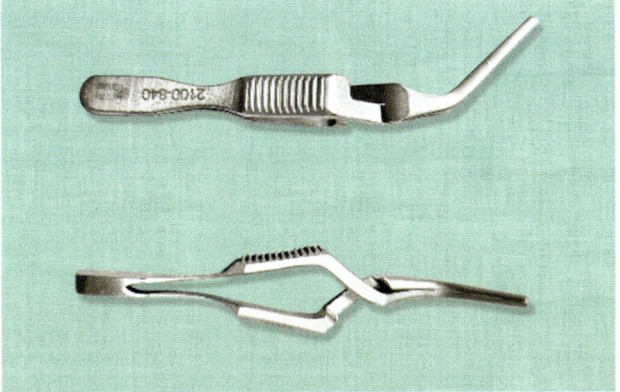

Fig. 8: Bulldog artery clamps.

- Compression over vein by mop till instruments and ligature are arranged.
- Clamping the ends of injured rent by vascular clamp: Bulldog clamp **(Fig. 8)**
- Repair the rent by continuous suture using 4-0 prolene.

Answer 12.3

In order to prevent DVT, LMWH 60 unit should be given daily subcutaneously arround the umbilicus in the immediate postoperative period for 5 days.

Question 13

A patient with stage IB2 CC, underwent radical hysterectomy with pelvic lymphadenectomy. Postoperatively, the histopathology report revealed the following:
- *Histology subtype:* Squamous cell carcinoma
- *Histology grade:* Grade II
- *Primary tumor diameter:* 2 × 3.2 cm
- *LVSI:* (+)
- *Surgical margin:* (+)
- *Two (right) and one (left) pelvic lymph nodes:* Metastatic
- *Parametrium:* Free of tumor
- *Cervical thickness:* >⅔ involved

   13.1. Enlist intermediate and high-risk factors, two for each from the above histopathology report. (0.5 × 4 = 2)

   13.2. Which adjuvant treatment should the patient receive postoperatively? (1)

   13.3. Is vaginal brachytherapy indicated in such a case? Give reasons. (1 + 0.5 × 2 = 2)

Answer 13.1

Intermediate risk factors:
- LVSI (+)
- Deep stromal invasion

High risk factors:
- Surgical margin (+) for malignancy
- Pelvic lymph nodes metastatic

Answer 13.2

Concurrent chemoradiation because there are two high-risk factors.

Answer 13.3

Vaginal brachytherapy **(Fig. 9)** is indicated here.

This is because the patient has:
- Positive surgical margin
- Deep stromal invasion

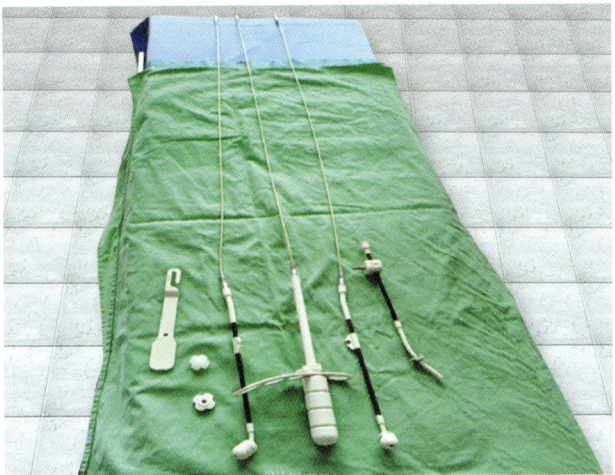

Fig. 9: Tandem, ovoid, and catheter tube for brachytherapy.

Question 14

An elderly woman was diagnosed with stage IIB CC. She was offered CCRT which is considered as the standard treatment. The patient wanted to know the details of treatment.

14.1. What is meant by CCRT? (1 × 2 = 2)

14.2. Specify the targeted coverage area in external beam radiotherapy (EBRT) and intracavitary brachytherapy (ICRT). (1 × 2 = 2)

14.3. If it is not feasible to give ICRT because of distorted anatomy, what is the next option? (1)

Answer 14.1

Concurrent chemoradiation means to administer chemotherapy and radiotherapy simultaneously.
- Chemotherapy regimen is once weekly intravenous (IV) cisplatin along with EBRT for 5 weeks.
- Radiotherapy includes EBRT 25 fractions in 5 weeks and ICRT three to five applications. The overall treatment time (OTT) is 55–56 days. ICRT is given within this time and thus is started during the last 2 weeks of EBRT.

Answer 14.2

External beam radiotherapy (Fig. 10A): It covers the cervix (tumor bed) and draining pelvic lymph node area. A dose of 40–50 Gy is usually given over abdomen in 5 weeks.

Intracavitary brachytherapy (Fig. 10B): It delivers high central dose to cervix (primary tumor) and reduced doses to the parametrium. A dose of 30–40 Gy is given in three to five fractions through vaginal route.

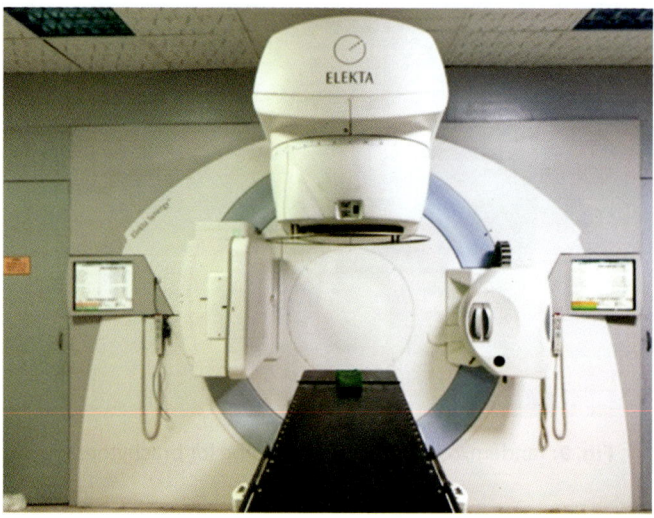

Fig. 10A: Linear accelerator machine for external beam radiotherapy (EBRT).

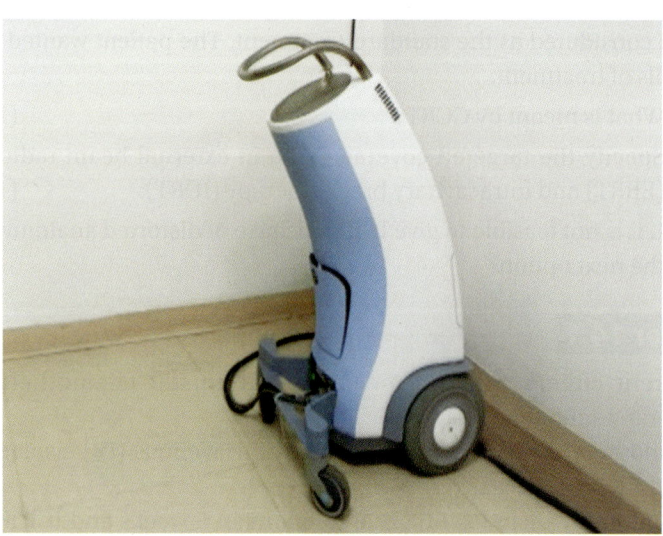

Fig. 10B: High dose rate (HDR) brachytherapy used for intracavitary brachytherapy.

Answer 14.3

Interstitial brachytherapy should be considered where multiple needles are inserted into the primary tumor and parametrium in situations where ICRT application is not possible due to vaginal stenosis.

Question 15

A 67-year-old lady underwent radical hysterectomy with pelvic lymphadenectomy for stage IB1 CC. Postoperatively histopathological evaluation revealed.
- *Surgical margin:* Negative.
- *Pelvic lymph nodes:* Reactive
- *PTD:* (2 × 3.5) cm
- *LVSI:* Positive
- *Cervical stromal invasion:* >⅔

15.1. Which adjunct treatment is suitable in this situation? Give reasons for such selection. (1 + 1 = 2)

15.2. What are the components of postoperative radiotherapy (PORT)? What benefit will be achieved? (0.5 × 2 + 1 = 2)

15.3. If no further treatment after radical hysterectomy is given in the above patient, mention two common sites of recurrence. (1)

Answer 15.1

Postoperative radiotherapy is the only suitable adjunct treatment.

Reasons for selection are:
Patient is node negative but intermediate risk features are present in primary tumor like:
- *LVSI:* Positive
- *Cervical stromal invasion:* >⅔

Answer 15.2

- PORT includes EBRT as standard protocol. In some situations, brachytherapy is added with EBRT.
  In the above scenario, there is deep cervical stromal invasion. ICRT in the form of brachytherapy can be added with EBRT.
- There will be significant reduction in risk of recurrence causing improvement in disease-free survival and OS.

Answer 15.3

80–90% of recurrences are seen in the central pelvis which includes vaginal vault and paravaginal soft tissue.

Question 16

A patient who is diagnosed as cancer cervix stage IIB is scheduled for CCRT. She is thoroughly counseled about the details of CCRT.

16.1. What are the preventable morbidities of conventional radiotherapy about which the patient should be counseled? (1.5)

16.2. Which new technique can reduce the morbidities and how? (1 + 1.5 = 2.5)

16.3. What is the ultimate goal of this new technique? (1)

Answer 16.1

There is late morbidity to the small bowel, rectum, urinary bladder, and vagina in the form of:
- Radiation proctitis
- Urgency of urine
- Sexual dysfunction

The patient should be informed about these complications before radiotherapy is started.

Answer 16.2

Intensity modulated radiotherapy (IMRT) **(Fig. 11)** use can reduce the above morbidities by undergoing 360° rotation and intensity modulation of radiation to organ at risk (OAR). In other words, IMRT distributes high radiation doses to the target organs evenly with better dose sparing of small bowel, rectum, and urinary bladder, thus reducing the toxicities.

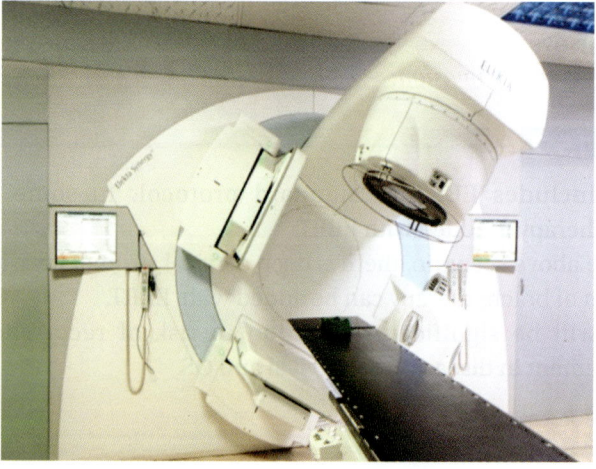

Fig. 11: Linear accelerator machine with intensity-modulated radiotherapy (IMRT) facility.

Answer 16.3

The ultimate goal of IMRT is to provide high-radiation dose to primary tumor with minimum toxicity and achieve prolong PFS and OS.

Question 17

A 27-year-old lady desiring fertility reported with cancer cervix which was clinically staged as stage IA1. The histopathology of cervical biopsy revealed squamous cell carcinoma, grade II with no LVSI and depth of invasion is 1.5 mm. In MRI of the abdomen, there was no involvement of endocervix, parametrium, and neither metastasis of pelvic lymph nodes were evident.

17.1 Justify the feasibility of fertility sparing treatment (FST) in this patient. Outline the different FST options. (2 + 1 = 3)

17.2. Is laparoscopy feasible in such situation? Enumerate the stepwise approach in such option. (0.5 + 1.5 = 2)

Answer 17.1

Justification for FST:
- The stage is IA1, grade II.
- No involvement of endocervix, para-aortic, and pelvic lymph nodes.
- No LVSI.
- Cervical stromal invasion is only 1.5 cm.

Fertility sparing treatment options are:
- Radical trachelectomy with pelvic lymphadenectomy
- Cone biopsy with pelvic lymphadenectomy

Answer 17.2

Laparoscopy is feasible in such situation.

Stepwise approach includes:
- Laparoscopic pelvic lymphadenectomy is done first followed by
- Radical vaginal trachelectomy which is done by open method.

Question 18

A young woman desiring fertility, reported with a histopathology report of loop electrodiathermy excisional procedure (LEEP) specimen revealing squamous cell carcinoma which has invaded <3 mm depth of cervical stroma. She is worried and wants standard treatment.

18.1. What is the stage of the disease? If LVSI is positive, what will be the treatment plan? (1 + 0.75 × 2 = 2.5)
18.2. Why pelvic lymphadenectomy is essential here? (1)
18.3. Enlist the components of specimen that should be included in cone biopsy. (0.5 × 3 = 1.5)

Answer 18.1

- The stage is IA1.
- Since the woman desires fertility, she may be offered any one of the following:
    - Cervical conization with pelvic lymphadenectomy
    - Radical trachelectomy with pelvic lymphadenectomy

Answer 18.2

Lymphovascular space invasion is an important prognostic indicator. When LVSI is positive, the likelihood of lymph node metastasis increases. As such, pelvic lymphadenectomy should be done.

Answer 18.3

Cone biopsy **(Fig. 12)** should include:
- Portion of ectocervix
- External os with entire transformation zone
- Endocervical canal with varying amount of deep tissues

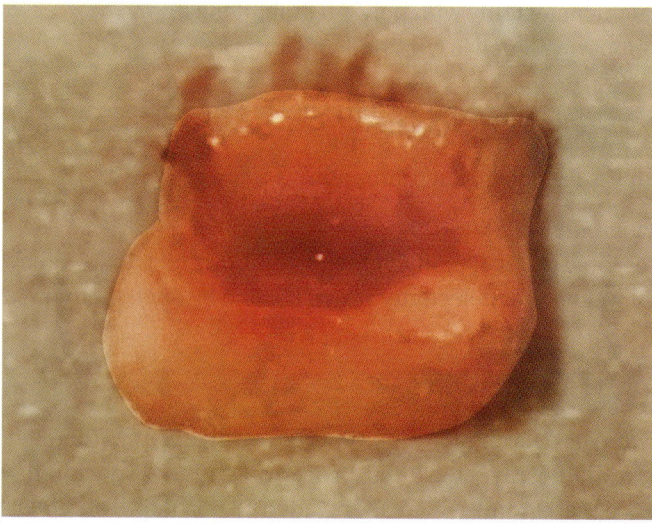

Fig. 12: Cone biopsy specimen of cervix.

Question 19

A 28-year-old lady was diagnosed with squamous cell carcinoma of cervix, stage IA1 by colposcopy-guided biopsy. She opted for fertility preservation surgery and came to cancer center for treatment.

19.1. What will be the next step for evaluation? Justify. $(0.5 \times 3 = 1.5)$

19.2. What are the treatment options for the patient? $(1 \times 3 = 3)$

19.3. Enumerate the follow up procedure if the patient is kept under observation. (0.5)

Answer 19.1

- Next step for evaluation is cold knife conization (CKC).
- The rationality of doing CKC is to:
  - Confirm the stage from depth of invasion
  - Determine histologic subtype, grade, margin status, and LVSI.

Answer 19.2

Fertility preservation treatment options for this patient includes:
- Only observation when surgical margins are negative and there in no LVSI. CKC will serve the therapeutic purpose then.
- Radical trachelectomy and pelvic lymphadenectomy if surgical margins are negative but LVSI is positive.
- If surgical margins are positive but LVSI is absent, repeat conization or radical trachelectomy.

Answer 19.3

Follow-up procedure in observation includes:
- Cytology
- Colposcopy
- ECC

Question 20

A 40-year-old lady was diagnosed as squamous cell carcinoma of cervix at 28 weeks of gestation. The stage at diagnosis was stage IB1. She consulted with her obstetrician and expressed her desire for continuation of pregnancy.

20.1. What will be its impact on prognosis if treatment is delayed? When should she deliver? $(1 + 0.5 = 1.5)$

20.2. Justify which mode of delivery is preferred. $(0.5 + 1 = 1.5)$

20.3. When definitive treatment will be planned? What complications will be encountered? $(1 + 1 = 2)$

Answer 20.1

There is no negative impact on prognosis compared with nonpregnant controls as found in evidence.

Pregnancy is continued up to 34 weeks of gestation until fetal lung maturity is achieved and then terminated.

Answer 20.2

The preferred mode of delivery is cesarean section because vaginal delivery is considered as the most significant predictor of recurrence as evident in literature.

Answer 20.3

Definite treatment is done at the same time when cesarean section is performed.

The complications that will be encountered are:
- Excessive blood loss during surgery
- Postoperative fever

Question 21

A 36-year-old lady was diagnosed as stage IIB squamous cell carcinoma at 16 weeks of gestation. The patient visited the hospital to get information about the impact of pregnancy on disease and treatment.

21.1. What specific information should be delivered to the patient during counseling? (1.5)
21.2. Enumerate the plan of treatment. (1.5)
21.3. Explain the role of neoadjuvant chemotherapy here. (1 + 1 = 2)

Answer 21.1

In this situation, definitive treatment for CC should be done without delay to avoid risk of progression because there will be a long waiting period of minimum 18 weeks (16 + 18 = 34 weeks) for the fetus to attain lung maturity and during this time, the disease will progress rapidly and thus treatment should be started immediately.

This information must be delivered to the patient during counseling.

Answer 21.2

The standard of treatment for stage IIB is to give chemoradiation with the fetus in situ.

During the first few fractions of radiation, there will be spontaneous abortion of conceptus following which the remaining fractions can be given smoothly.

Answer 21.3

- Neoadjuvant chemotherapy (NACT) is planned to prevent disease progression in woman with locally advanced CC if she desires pregnancy continuation.
- The standard regimen is platinum-based chemotherapy which is given from 14 weeks gestational age onward and is safe both for the mother and the fetus, but the impact of treatment delay on survival is not well studied.

Question 22

A 47-year-old multiparous lady was diagnosed as stage IB3 CC. She was admitted in a tertiary care center for treatment.

22.1. Which one is the preferred treatment option among the following? Give reason for such preference. (1 + 2 = 3)
- Primary chemoradiation
- NACT followed by radical hysterectomy
- Radical hysterectomy followed by adjuvant radiation
- Chemoradiation followed by extrafascial hysterectomy

22.2. Can IMRT replace traditional radiation in such situation if lymph nodes are unresectable? (2)

Answer 22.1

The preferred treatment option is primary chemoradiation.

The standard protocol is cisplatin once weekly along with EBRT: 45–50 Gy for rest of the 5 days in a week for 5 weeks.

ICRT is given in three to five applications: 30–35 Gy anytime from last 2 weeks of EBRT at an interval of 7–10 days.

Reasons of preference:
- Carcinoma cervix IB3 means bulky tumor which is associated with high incidence of central recurrence, pelvic, and para-aortic lymph node metastasis and distant metastasis.
- Primary chemoradiation will effectively control such predicted outcome and simultaneously will avoid adverse morbidity associated with dual modality of treatment that is surgery followed by radiotherapy.
- The ultimate outcome will be improved PFS and OS.

Answer 22.2

Conventional radiation is associated with increased toxicity. In such situation, IMRT is able to safely deliver high doses of radiation to tumor site and lymph node area while limiting the dose of radiation to highly proliferating normal tissue such as bowel, bladder, and vagina.

There is higher rate of tumor response and at the same time, lower gastrointestinal tract (GIT) and vaginal toxicities.

Thus, there is improvement in PFD and OS.

Question 23

A woman who underwent radical hysterectomy for carcinoma cervix IB1 is found to have no urine in the urine bag 6 hours after the surgery.

23.1. Enumerate four measures that should be taken immediately. (0.5 × 4 = 2)
23.2. Which imaging can detect ureteric injury accurately? (1)
23.3. If the left ureter is injured at its distal third producing a rent of 0.5 cm, what will be the management? (2)

Answer 23.1

- Enquire whether the urine bag was emptied without keeping record.
- Assess vital parameters, level of dehydration, and urine color.
- Assess whether the urinary bladder is distended or not.
- Flush the catheter with distilled water to remove blood clot.
- Hydrate the patient with 200–300 mL IV fluid in 1 hour and observe the urine output.

Answer 23.2

A CT urogram (CT of the abdomen and the pelvis with IV contrast and delayed image) can accurately identify ureteral injury.

Answer 23.3

- Since the rent in the ureter is small, ureteral double J stent insertion and keeping it in situ for 21 days is the first line treatment.
- If spontaneous healing fails to occur, repair the ureteric rent by open method keeping the stent in situ.

Question 24

A 48-year-old obese woman is scheduled for radical hysterectomy for CC stage IB1. The woman's family is concerned about surgical site infection (SSI) and have requested to take all protective measures to minimize the risk.

24.1. Define surgical site infection. Enlist the causative agents responsible for SSI. (1 + 1 = 2)

24.2. Enlist six best practices you will adopt to reduce SSI. (0.5 × 6 = 3)

Answer 24.1

Definition: Surgical site infection is defined as infection occurring up to 30 days after surgery and affecting either the incision or deep tissue at the operation site.

Causative agents: The responsible pathogens originate from patients endogenous flora.

Commonly seen pathogens are:
- *Staphylococcus*
- Coagulase-negative *Staphylococcus*
- *Enterococcus* spp.
- *Escherichia coli*

Answer 24.2

Six best practices to reduce SSI
1. IV antibiotics should be administered 60 minutes before skin incision.
2. The antibiotic should have a longer half-life and broad spectrum coverage such as cefazolin and cefoxitin.
3. The dose should be repeated if the operation time is prolonged beyond 3 hours or when blood loss is >1,000 mL.
4. The dose should be doubled for woman >70 kg weight.
5. Hair clipping is preferred for hair removal before surgery if it is mandatory.
6. Chlorhexidine-alcohol is preferred over povidone-iodine.

Question 25

An obese elderly woman who is a known case of hypertension and diabetes mellitus underwent radical hysterectomy. On the 4th postoperative day, the patient complained of throbbing pain at the wound area with mild fever. On inspection, there was redness, swelling, and discharge from one end of the wound.

25.1. What immediate action should be undertaken? (0.5 × 3 = 1.5)

25.2. Identify three factors which contributed in the impairment of wound healing. (0.5 × 3 = 1.5)

25.3. When will wound closure be done if wound disruption has occurred? How wound healing will now take place? (1 + 1 = 2)

Answer 25.1

- Two or three stitches at the red, swollen area of the wound should be cut and pus is drained out.
- The pus is sent for culture sensitivity.
- Antibiotic should be changed according to the culture sensitivity report.

Answer 25.2

Three factors which contributed in the impairment of wound healing:
1. Old age
2. Obesity
3. Diabetes mellitus

Answer 25.3

- Secondary closure will be done when:
  - Infection subsides
  - Wound is filled up from the base
- Wound healing will take place by formation of granulation tissue from the base.

Question 26

A 43-year-old lady underwent primary radical hysterectomy for early-stage CC. 8 months after surgery, the patient reported sexual dysfunction.

26.1. What is the prevalence of sexual dysfunction following radical hysterectomy? Why it happens? $(1 + 0.5 \times 2 = 2)$

26.2. What prophylactic measures can overcome the sexual dysfunction problem? $(1 + 1 = 2)$

26.3. Which modality of treatment causes more sexual dysfunction and why? $(0.5 \times 2 = 1)$

Answer 26.1

- Among CC survivors, sexual dysfunction is reported in 55% patients treated by radical hysterectomy.
- Sexual dysfunction following surgery is due to any of the following: They may remain alone or in combination:
  - Insufficient lubrication or dry vagina
  - Reduced vaginal length and elasticity

Answer 26.2

- In premenopausal women, resection of vagina in radical hysterectomy should be limited within 1.5 cm.
- Nerve sparing radical hysterectomy should be practiced frequently.

Answer 26.3

Sexual dysfunction is more pronounced following primary radiotherapy than primary surgery because of:
- Vaginal atrophy
- Fibrosis
- Stenosis

Question 27

A 67-year-old lady with CC underwent radical hysterectomy 8 hours back. Her left calf was found to be swollen with tenderness and pitting edema.

27.1. Enlist the clinical features in the scenario that goes in favor of DVT. (0.5 × 5 = 2.5)

27.2. Which two investigatory tools are needed to confirm the diagnosis? (0.5 × 2 = 1)

27.3. What specific treatment should be offered to the patient? (1.5)

Answer 27.1

TABLE 2: Clinical features suggesting deep vein thrombosis (DVT) with scoring.

Clinical features	Score
Malignancy—cervical cancer	1
Radical hysterectomy (major surgery)	1
<12 hours back	1
Calf swollen	1
Local tenderness	1
Pitting edema	1
Total Score	**6**

The score between 3 and 8 indicates the high probability of DVT.

Answer 27.2

Two investigatory tools to confirm diagnosis are:
1. Compression USG showing blood clot in ileo-saphenous-popliteal vein
2. Age-adjusted D-dimer positive in blood

Answer 27.3

Low molecular weight heparin (LMWH) **(Fig. 13)** subcutaneously is given for 5 days followed by oral anticoagulant or warfarin for minimum 3 months.

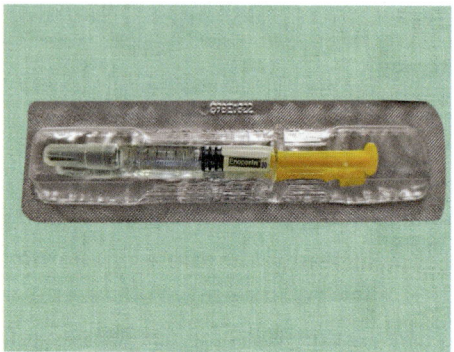

Fig. 13: Low molecular weight heparin.

Question 28

Conventional radiation therapy is usually given in a fractionated course with daily doses of 180–200 CGy per fraction in cancer cervix.

28.1. Why is fractionated irradiation important? (1)

28.2. When are the cells most sensitive and resistant to radiation in fractionated course? (1 + 1 = 2)

28.3. How hyperfractionated strategy is helpful in advanced stage CC? (2)

Answer 28.1

Fractionated irradiation permits recovery or maximum repair of sublethal injury of normal tissue and tumor.

Answer 28.2

- Cells are most sensitive to radiation in late G2 phase and during mitosis of cell cycle.
- Cells are most resistant to radiation in mid to late S phase and early G1 phase of cell cycle.

Answer 28.3

In advanced stage CC, primary radiation therapy in the form of EBRT with brachytherapy is the gold standard. Hyperfractionated strategy here decreases the expected late morbidity to the bowel, bladder, and vaginal vault.

CHAPTER 4

Endometrial Carcinoma

Question 1

A 40-year-old lady reports with intermenstrual bleeding. Transvaginal sonography (TVS) reveals an endometrial mass (2 × 3) cm arising from the posterior wall of the uterus with no invasion in myometrium. She is advised for endometrial sampling.

1.1. What are three different ways by which endometrial sampling can be done? (0.5 × 3 = 1.5)

1.2. Which method of endometrial sampling is best? Give five important reasons. (1 + 0.5 × 5 = 3.5)

Answer 1.1

Methods of endometrial sampling are:
1. Endometrial biopsy
2. Dilatation and curettage (D&C)
3. Hysteroscopic-guided sampling which is gold standard

Answer 1.2

Hysteroscopic endometrial sampling is the best method because:
1. Hysteroscopy provides an accurate evaluation of the endometrial cavity by direct vision and allows accurate sampling of suspected lesion.
2. Other endometrial pathology such as polyp can be excluded.
3. Hysteroscopy is accurate in assessment of cervical involvement.
4. It serves therapeutic purpose in young woman who wants to preserve fertility.
5. Achieves better outcome in infertility with less recurrence.

Question 2

A 68-year-old lady was diagnosed with endometrial cancer on endometrial sampling. She was advised for further evaluation.

2.1. Enlist five important information you must know preoperatively to plan treatment. (0.5 × 5 = 2.5)

2.2. Which two imaging tools will you select for preoperative evaluation? (0.5 × 2 = 1)

2.3. What information will magnetic resonance imaging (MRI) provide for preoperative staging? (1.5)

Answer 2.1

Five important information that must be known preoperatively are:
1. Histologic type
2. Histologic grade
3. Depth of myometrial invasion
4. Cervical stromal involvement
5. Extrauterine spread of disease in—adnexa, omentum, and pelvic and para-aortic lymph nodes.

Answer 2.2

For preoperative evaluation, the two important imaging tools are:
1. TVS
2. MRI of pelvis and lower abdomen

Answer 2.3

Magnetic resonance imaging will provide information on:
- Depth of myometrial invasion
- Cervical stromal involvement
- Extent of extrauterine metastasis—pelvic lymph node, ovaries, and omentum.

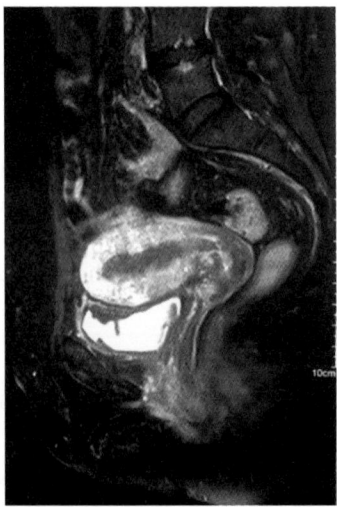

Fig. 1: MRI of pelvis showing endometrial carcinoma confined within endometrium.

Endometrial Carcinoma

Magnetic resonance imaging shows endometrial growth is superficial with no invasion into the myometrium. Cervical stromal involvement is absent and no extra uterine spread **(Fig. 1)**.

Question 3

A 42-year-old lady came with the complaint of intermenstrual bleeding for last 6 months. She wanted a thorough evaluation for diagnosis.

3.1. Name four investigations which are accepted for evaluation of endometrial pathology. (0.25 × 4 = 1)
3.2. Why fractional curettage is not randomly done for evaluation nowadays? (1 × 2 = 2)
3.3. Which investigation is the most cost-effective and safe in endometrial sampling? Compare it with pipelle. (0.5 + 0.5 × 3 = 2)

Answer 3.1

1. D&C
2. Fractional curettage
3. Hysteroscopic-guided endometrial sampling
4. Endometrial sampling by Endo sampler:
   a. Pipelle
   b. Endometrial suction kit

Answer 3.2

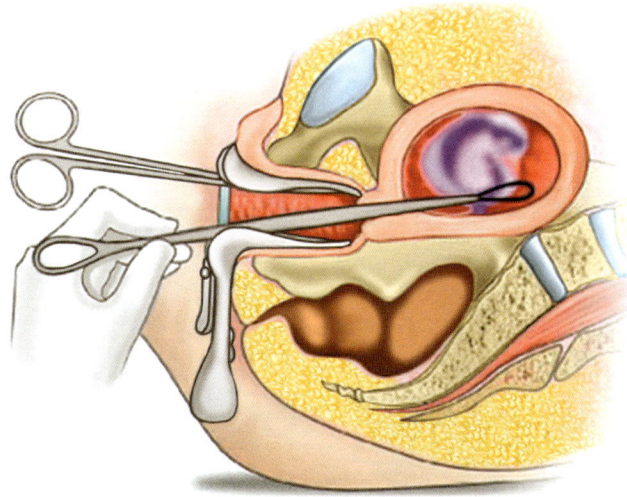

Fig. 2: Fractional curettage.

Fractional curettage (**Fig. 2**) is not randomly done nowadays because:
- Endometrial cancer is now staged surgically which can differentiate stage 1 from stage 2.
- Advancement in MRI has made easy to rule out cervical involvement.

Answer 3.3

The cost-effective and safe investigation for endometrial sampling is endometrial suction kit.

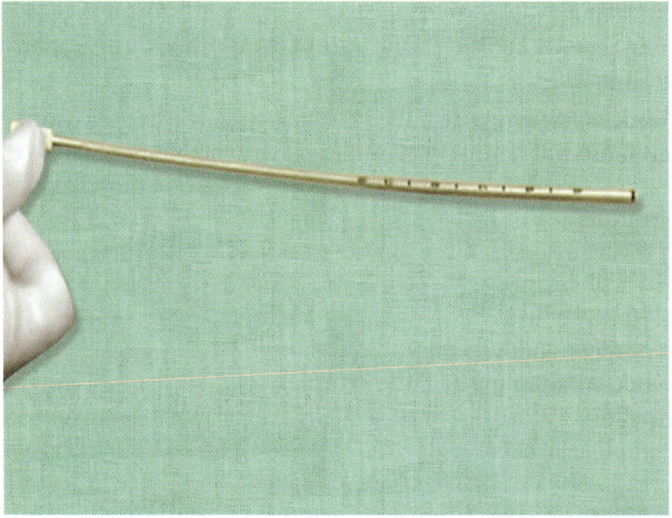

Fig. 3A: Pipelle.

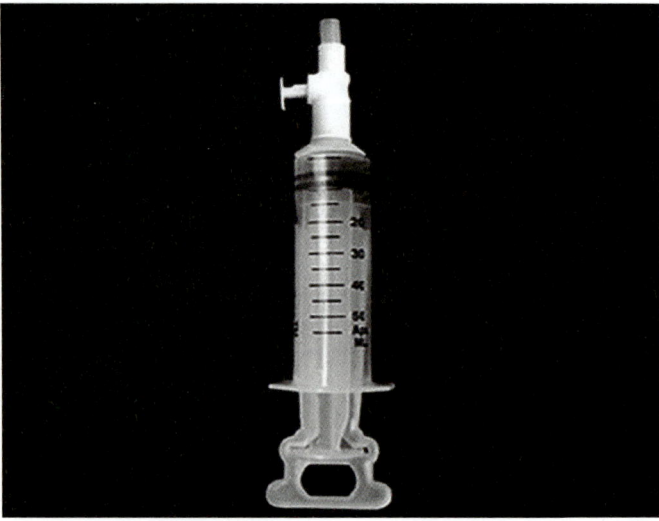

Fig. 3B: Endometrial suction kit.

TABLE 1: Comparison between pipelle and endometrial suction kit.

	Pipelle (Fig. 3A)	Endometrial suction kit (Fig. 3B)
Adequacy of tissue	Insufficient tissue is obtained	Sufficient tissue is obtained
Acceptance	Not good	Good
Diagnostic yield	Not reliable	Reliable

Question 4

A 38-year-old obese lady reported with intermittent bleeding for the last 2 months. Endometrial sampling revealed atypical hyperplasia/endometrial intraepithelial neoplasia (EIN) **(Fig. 4)**. TVS revealed normal genital organs.

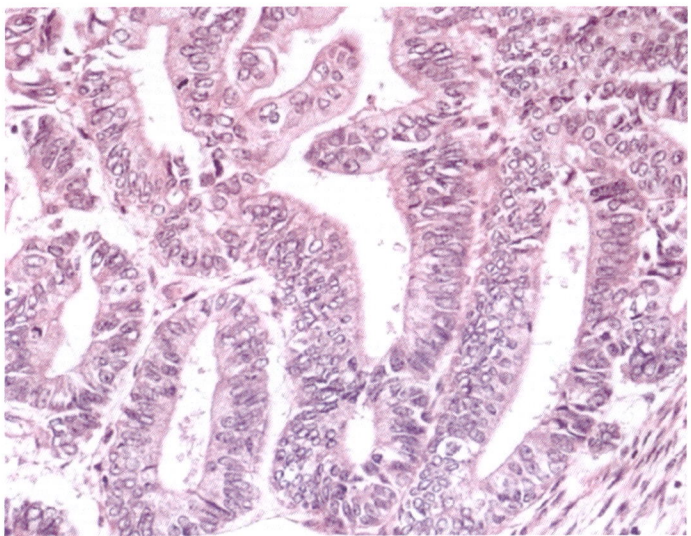

Fig. 4: Endometrial intraepithelial neoplasia (microscopic view).

4.1. What is the clinical significance of EIN? (1)
4.2. Which factor contributes to EIN and how? (1 + 1 = 2)
4.3. Name the curative treatment. What additional benefit is obtained from the treatment? (1 + 0.5 × 2 = 2)

Answer 4.1

Endometrial intraepithelial neoplasia is the direct precursor of endometrial cancer. 40% of women with EIN diagnosis will develop endometrial carcinoma (EC) within 1 year. Those who will not develop cancer within a year, there will be 45-fold increased risk of future EC.

Answer 4.2

Obesity is the contributing factor.

There is peripheral conversion of androgen to estrogen by aromatase in fat causing endometrial hyperplasia.

Answer 4.3

Hysterectomy is the curative treatment.

The additional benefit obtained from hysterectomy is:
- Uterus is available to confirm the diagnosis and exclude the coexistence of carcinoma.
- It acts as a definitive preventive strategy for cancer.

Question 5

A 32-year-old lady who has been diagnosed as having atypical hyperplasia/endometrial intraepithelial neoplasia (EIN) wants conservative treatment. A thorough investigation has excluded invasive carcinoma. She wants to have a trial for future pregnancy.

5.1. Which three types of progesterone can be offered to her?

$(0.5 \times 3 = 1.5)$

5.2. Which progestin is the preferred option for her? (1)

5.3. Briefly outline the two concerns about which the patient must be informed before starting progestin. $(1 + 1.5 = 2.5)$

Answer 5.1

1. Medroxyprogesterone acetate (MPA)
2. Megestrol acetate
3. Levonorgestrel intrauterine device (LNG-IUD)

Answer 5.2

- Since the woman is young, MPA will be preferred.
- LNG-IUD is a newer option and meta-analysis has shown better efficacy than other progestins.

Answer 5.3

This is not a standard treatment for EIN, because:
1. The risk of malignant transformation to carcinoma is high (25–50%).
2. The possibility of a co-existent carcinoma in EIN persists ranging from 10 to 40%.

Question 6

A 67-year-old nulliparous lady presents with recurrent postmenopausal bleeding due to a small EC which has escaped diagnosis by D&C. Her current diagnosis was made by hysteroscopic-directed biopsy **(Fig. 5)**.

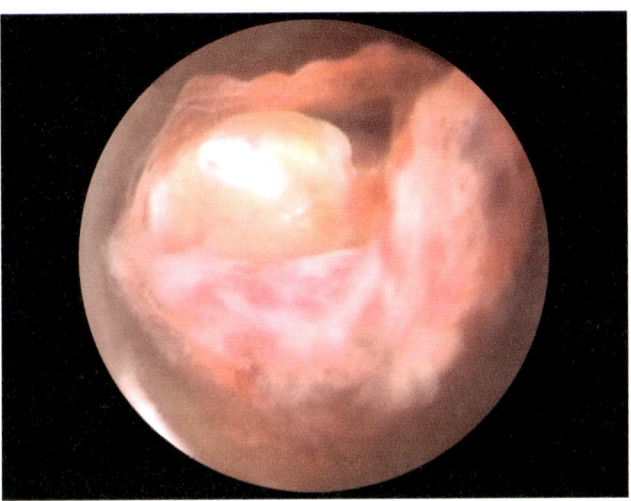

Fig. 5: Intracavitary lesion viewed by hysteroscope.

6.1. Why hysteroscopic-directed biopsy was able to diagnose endometrial cancer while D&C failed? (2)
6.2. What is the disadvantage of using hysteroscopy in EC? (1.5)
6.3. What is the limitation of using hysteroscopy in EC? (1.5)

Answer 6.1

Hysteroscopic-directed biopsy is considered superior than blunt curettage in diagnosing EC because:
- The panoramic view of hysteroscopy identifies the location of focal EC from where directed biopsy can be obtained. Thus, accuracy for diagnosing EC is highest (99.5%).
- Hysteroscopy-directed biopsy can determine the tumor grade with an accuracy of 97%.

Answer 6.2

The distension of the uterus by fluid may cause tumor cell dissemination through the fallopian tube into the peritoneal cavity worsening the prognosis of the disease. But evidence has shown that it does not increase intra-abdominal tumor dissemination neither it alters the tumor stage or worsen prognosis.

Answer 6.3

Depth of myometrial invasion cannot be assessed by hysteroscope. Thus, accurate staging of EC is difficult.

Question 7

A 44-year-old lady who has been diagnosed as endometrioid EC grade 2 is admitted for management. She underwent surgical treatment.

7.1. What surgical treatment is recommended for her? (1)
7.2. Why is it essential to remove ovaries in such a condition? (0.5 × 3 = 1.5)
7.3. Which histological features after surgery will suggest low-risk endometrial cancer? (0.5 × 5 = 2.5)

Answer 7.1

The recommended surgical treatment is total abdominal hysterectomy with bilateral salpingo-oophorectomy (BSO) **(Fig. 6)** with surgical staging.

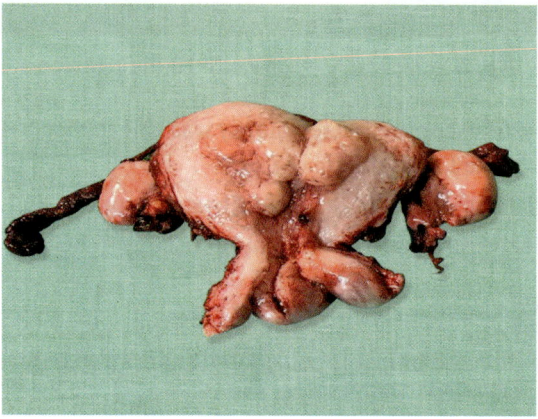

Fig. 6: Resected uterus with endometrial growth and both ovaries.

Answer 7.2

Both ovaries should be removed even if they appear normal because:
- They may contain micro-metastasis.
- They can harbor ovarian cancer concurrently.
- They are at increased risk for ovarian cancer in future.

Answer 7.3

Histological features suggesting low-risk endometrial cancer are:
- Histologic subtype—endometrioid

- Histologic grade—1–2
- Myometrial invasion <50%
- No cervical stromal involvement
- Lymphovascular space invasion (LVSI)—absent

Question 8

A 67-year-old postmenopausal lady was diagnosed with endometrial adenocarcinoma on a background of atrophic endometrium, endometrioid type grade 3 on D&C. MRI reveals >50% of myometrial involvement.

    8.1. What is the overall prognosis of the disease? Explain reasons. (3)

    8.2. What will be the treatment? (2)

Answer 8.1

The overall prognosis is poor because:
- Patient is in advanced age group.
- The tumor is grade 3 involving >50% of myometrium which has a propensity of high positive pelvic lymph node.
- These tumors have developed on atrophic endometrium which suggest that they are less hormone sensitive and generally more aggressive.

Answer 8.2

The treatment will be total abdominal hysterectomy, BSO, and pelvic and para-aortic lymphadenectomy with omentectomy.

Question 9

A 47-year-old lady with diabetes mellitus (DM) and hypertension is diagnosed as endometrioid type endometrial cancer **(Fig. 7)**. She reported to gynecologic oncologist and was counseled for risk stratification which is the primary plan of treatment.

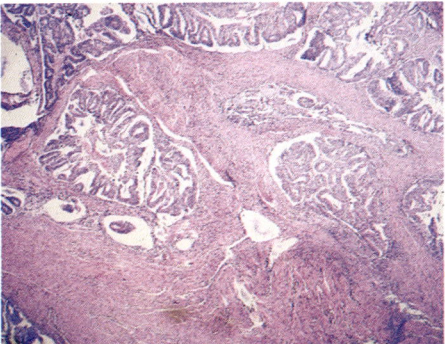

Fig. 7: Endometrioid type endometrial adenocarcinoma showing confluents glands lacking intervening stroma.

9.1. Enlist three important significance of risk stratification. (0.5 × 3 = 1.5)
9.2. How risk stratification will be done in this patient? (1.5 + 2 = 3.5)

Answer 9.1

Risk stratification in such a diagnosis is important to:
1. Determine the extent of surgery by categorizing the patient into low-risk, intermediate-risk, or high-risk group.
2. Plan adjuvant treatment.
3. Predict prognosis.

Answer 9.2

It will be done by:
- Endometrial biopsy by pipelle or curettage which is already done here. This will characterize:
    - Histologic type
    - Histologic grade and exclude
    - Cervical involvement
- Contrast-enhanced MRI to stage endometrial cancer preoperatively by assessing:
    - Depth of myometrial invasion
    - Cervical involvement
    - Metastatic spread of disease to pelvic, para-aortic lymph node, omentum, and colon

Question 10

According to current practice standards, the grading of endometrioid endometrial cancer is done by the International Federation of Gynaecology and Obstetrics (FIGO) grading.

10.1. What is the basis of FIGO grading? (1)
10.2. Enumerate the FIGO grading system. (2.5)
10.3. What is the importance of FIGO grading in endometrial cancer? (1.5)

Answer 10.1

The International Federation of Gynaecology and Obstetrics (FIGO) grading is based on the degree of glandular differentiation.

Answer 10.2

- Grade 1 tumor exhibits <5% solid, nonglandular, nonsquamous growth.
- Grade 2 tumor exhibits from 6 to 50% nonglandular, nonsquamous growth.
- Grade 3 tumor exhibits >50% nonglandular, nonsquamous growth.

Answer 10.3

It is used to provide prognostic information that can be used to guide the extent of surgery and use of adjuvant chemotherapy or radiation therapy.

Question 11

A 67-year-old postmenopausal lady was diagnosed on endometrial sampling as endometrial adenocarcinoma with atrophic endometrium. The histopathology was serous subtype, grade 3.

11.1. What other information could be obtained on histopathology? What is the impact of knowing the information? (1 + 1 = 2)

11.2. The prognosis of the disease as evident in the above scenario is poor. Justify. (3)

Answer 11.1

Hormone receptor status of endometrial cancer, i.e., whether the cancer is positive for one (estrogen or progesterone) or both receptors.

Patients who are positive for one or both receptors have longer survival than patients whose carcinoma lacks the corresponding receptors.

Answer 11.2

The prognosis is poor because of:
- The high-risk factors:
  - Age >60 years
  - Serous subtype
  - Grade 3
  - Atrophic endometrium
- These patients are diagnosed mostly in advanced stage, have quick extrauterine dissemination and frequent recurrence.
- They have deep myometrial invasion.
- LVSI positive.
- Lymph node metastasis.
- They are less hormone sensitive.

Thus, they have unfavorable prognosis with overall survival (OS) ranging between 40 and 60% at 5 years.

Question 12

A 67-year-old postmenopausal lady was diagnosed with serous adenocarcinoma of endometrium grade 2. MRI showed >50% of myometrial invasion.

12.1. Categorize the type of endometrial cancer. Specify the contribution of this type in incidence. (0.5 × 2 = 1)
12.2. What will be the standard treatment for such a patient? Justify the reliability of MRI in regards to depth of myometrial invasion after surgery. (1.5 + 0.5 = 2)
12.3. Justify that the disease has poor prognosis. (2)

Answer 12.1

- The patient belongs to type II endometrial cancer.
- Type II EC contributes only about 10% of EC incidence.

Answer 12.2

- *Surgery:* Total abdominal hysterectomy with BSO, omentectomy, pelvic, and para-aortic lymphadenectomy.
- *Adjuvant treatment:* Chemotherapy (paclitexel + carboplatin) with pelvic external beam radiation therapy (EBRT).

The myometrial invasion in resected uterus **(Fig. 8)** is normally found to correlate with MRI findings. Thus, MRI is reliable in this regards.

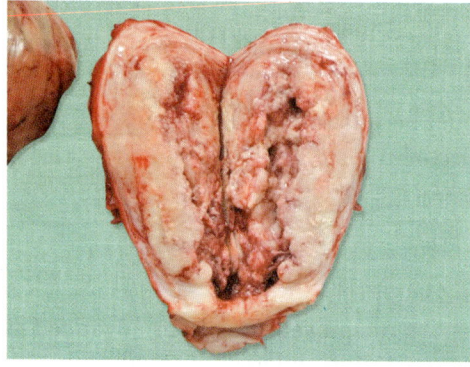

Fig. 8: Resected uterus with endometrial growth invading >50% myometrium.

Answer 12.3

Prognosis is poor.
- It is aggressive in nature and is diagnosed at advanced stage.
- Rapidly disseminating intra-abdominally (50%).
- Nonestrogen dependent.
- Myometrial invasion is >50% causing increased propensity for lymph node metastasis.
- High recurrence rate (50%)
- Low OS rate

Question 13

A 53-year-old postmenopausal lady, on evaluation, was found to have endometrioid type endometrial cancer, grade 1 with ovarian cancer.

13.1. What is the stage of the disease if the ovarian tumor is metastatic? (1)

13.2. How can you confirm that the ovarian tumor is metastatic? (1 + 1 = 2)

13.3. How will you treat the condition? (1 + 1 = 2)

Answer 13.1

Stage IIIA

Answer 13.2

- On histopathology, there will be similarity between two tumors.
- On immunohistochemistry (IHC), the ovarian tumor will show:
  - Estrogen receptor (ER) and/or progesterone receptor (PR) positivity
  - Bcl-2 negativity

Answer 13.3

Unless there is clear evidence that ovarian tumor is metastatic, each will be considered as primary lesion and treatment will be done accordingly.

The treatment should include:
- TAH + BSO + surgical staging
- Adjuvant chemotherapy depending on the stage of ovarian cancer

Question 14

Sentinel lymph node (SLN) biopsy is accepted as a standard approach with favorable results in some cancers.

14.1. Why is the concept of SLN biopsy established in the management of cancer? (2.5)

14.2. What is the role of SLN biopsy in endometrial cancer? (2.5)

Answer 14.1

Sentinel lymph node is a regional lymph node that drains directly the lymph from the primary tumor.
- It is considered the first lymph node to receive lymph borne metastatic cancer cells.

- It is also considered representative of other draining lymph nodes. So, if it is metastatic, one can easily understand the status of other lymph nodes and plan the extent of surgery.

Answer 14.2

Revised FIGO staging in 2009 has included pelvic and para-aortic lymphadenectomy as one of the most important prognostic factors in EC.

There is argument that lymphadenectomy increases the peroperative and postoperative complications and thus systemic lymphadenectomy is not necessary in women of low-risk group who are in early stage.

Women with negative SLN for metastasis can thus be managed by:

Sentinel lymph node biopsy instead of systemic lymph node biopsy, thereby reducing the morbidity.

Thus, SLN biopsy is indicated in early-stage endometrial cancer.

Question 15

A 43-year-old lady was diagnosed as endometrioid endometrial cancer grade 3. MRI revealed myometrial invasion >50%, but there was no cervical stromal involvement and lymphadenopathy **(Fig. 9)**. The lady was admitted for management.

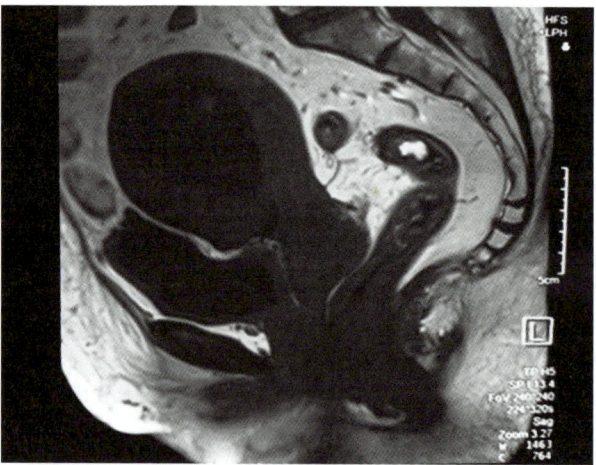

Fig. 9: Growth occupying whole endometrial cavity and invading >50% of myometrium.

15.1. What is the standard surgical treatment? (1.5)

15.2. Will lymphadenectomy be included in the surgical staging? Justify the answer. (1.5)

15.3. What information lymphadenectomy will provide? (2)

Answer 15.1

The standard surgical treatment is total abdominal hysterectomy, BSO, and complete surgical staging.

Answer 15.2

Lymphadenectomy will be included in the surgical staging of this patient because high-risk features are present here like:
- Grade 3 tumor
- >50% myometrial invasion

Answer 15.3

Lymphadenectomy will:
- Assign the surgical stage
- Provide therapeutic benefit in patients with positive nodes
- Stratify patients for adjuvant treatment
- Provide prognostic information

Question 16

A 40-year-old lady who deferred pregnancy for career building was diagnosed as endometrioid, endometrial cancer grade 1. She is unwilling to undergo surgery and has fulfilled all the criteria for fertility sparing treatment (FST).

16.1. Which treatment can be offered to her and for how long? (2)

16.2. Compare the offered treatment with other option, i.e., combined hysteroscopy and progesterone. (3)

Answer 16.1

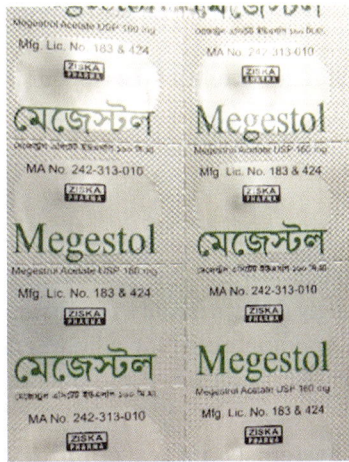

Fig. 10A: Megestrol acetate.

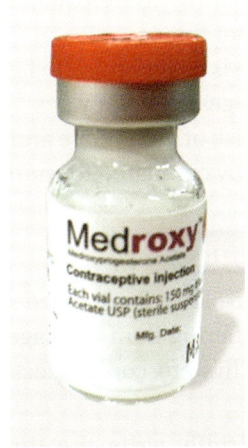

Fig. 10B: Medroxyprogesterone acetate.

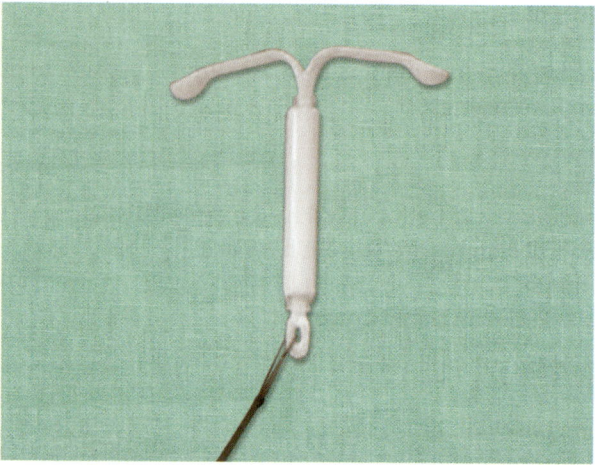

Fig. 10C: Levonorgestrel intrauterine device (LNG-IUD).

Progestin therapy is available in the form of following. Anyone can be offered:
- Medroxyprogesterone acetate (400–600 mg) **(Fig. 10A)**
- Megestrol acetate (160–320 mg) **(Fig. 10B)**
- LNG-IUD **(Fig. 10C)**

It should be continued for 6–9 months.

Answer 16.2

- Progestin therapy alone has only 50% response rate while combination of hysteroscopy and progesterone has 100% response rate indicating shorter time period to remission.
- The possibility of recurrence is high as the disease persists within the endometrium in spite of progesterone therapy, while the disease is resected by hysteroscope and progesterone is given on endometrium without tumor.
- There is faster return to fertility in combination while it takes longer time in progestin therapy.
- The risk of recurrence and progression of diseases is higher progesterone therapy compared to combination.

Question 17

A 40-year-old well-educated nullipara strongly desires fertility preservation. She is suffering from EC stage 1A, grade 1, endometrioid type. She wants to undergo hysteroscopic resection of EC after being counseled thoroughly on this issue.

17.1. Briefly write the three steps of hysteroscopic resection of EC.
(0.5 × 3 = 1.5)

17.2. What is the subsequent treatment following hysteroscopic resection? (0.5 × 3 = 1.5)

17.3. Which parameters following hysteroscopy will justify FST. (2)

Answer 17.1

Hysteroscopic resection is a three-step procedure.

Step 1: Removal of endometrial lesion

Step 2: Removal of 3–4 mm of underlying myometrium

Step 3: Removal of endometrium and myometrium surrounding the lesion

Answer 17.2

High progesterone therapy. Anyone of the following can be given:
- Medroxyprogesterone acetate
- Megestrol acetate
- LNG-IUD

Answer 17.3

After hysteroscopic resection, the tumor and underlying and surrounding tissue is subjected to pathologic analysis.

If the resected tumor is positive and adjacent endometrium and underlying myometrium is negative, it means EC is confined within endometrium without myometrial invasion. In other words, the resection margin is free. Thus, FST in the form of progesterone can be given.

Question 18

A 40-year-old recently married lady was diagnosed with endometrial cancer, endometroid type, G1. She fulfilled all the criteria for conservative treatment and accordingly she was given progesterone therapy for fertility preservation.

18.1. How will the patient be monitored during the treatment? (0.5 × 2 = 1)

18.2. What will be the surveillance after treatment? (2.5)

18.3. What is the outcome of treatment? (0.5 × 3 = 1.5)

Answer 18.1

The patient's monitoring during treatment includes:
- Endometrial sampling every 3 months to assess the response of treatment
- Further evaluation with MRI is done after 6 months

Answer 18.2

Surveillance after treatment includes:
- Endometrial sampling every 3 months after progestin cessation. If negative for malignancy on 2 occasions the patient is declared as complete remission. Thereafter, the patient is encouraged to seek pregnancy advice from infertility specialists. Most cases conceive with assisted reproductive technology (ART).
- But if there is stable or progressive disease, patient is advised for definitive surgery.

Answer 18.3

The response rate following FST is approximately 75%.

The recurrence rate ranges between 30 and 40%.

Overall pregnancy rate is 30–35% but 18–20% need ART.

Question 19

A 38-year-old lady was diagnosed with endometrial cancer. Her mother died at the age of 48 years with the same disease.

19.1. Which specific investigation should be done in this lady? Give reasons. (0.5 + 1.5 = 2)

19.2. How it will be done and what is its objective? (1.5 + 1.5 = 3)

Answer 19.1

Tumor testing for genetic risk assessment should be done in this lady.

The reasons are:
- 3–5% of EC is caused by inherited predisposition.
- Lynch syndrome or hereditary nonpolyposis colorectal cancer (HNPCC) accounts for the majority of inherited predisposition.

Answer 19.2

Tumor testing will include:
- IHC of formalin fixed paraffin embedded tissue to detect one of the four mismatched repair (MMR) proteins—MLH1, MSH2, MSH6, and PNS2, which are responsible for causing Lynch syndrome.
- *Microsatellite instability (MSI)* analysis using both tumor and normal tissue to determine tumor phenotype of deficient DNA repair.

   This patient is at significant life-time risk of developing a second primary malignancy either in the ovary or the colon.

Question 20

Both mother and daughter had endometrial cancer which was diagnosed between the 4th to 5th decades of their life. After completion of treatment, the daughter was worried and she repeatedly visited her physician for checkup.

20.1. If the lady belongs to Lynch syndrome on tumor testing, what will be its implication? (2)
20.2. Enumerate the expected nature of EC in this patient. (2)
20.3. If the lady has a sister, what would be the advice for her? (1)

Answer 20.1

- The lady must undergo appropriate colon and ovarian cancer screening after completion of standard treatment for endometrial cancer.
- Other relevant family members including sister should also undergo targeted genetic testing for the same mutation.

Answer 20.2

The EC in this lady has the probability of being diagnosed in stage I. The histology might be anyone of the three subtypes—endometrioid, serous, and clear cell. The tumor may arise from lower uterine segment.

Answer 20.3

The sister should undergo risk reducing hysterectomy and salpingo-oophorectomy after the family is complete as there is risk of endometrial and ovarian cancer.

Question 21

A 42-year-old lady was treated for breast cancer. She is on tamoxifen therapy **(Fig. 11)** and has been thoroughly counseled on the issue. She is worried and has come to gynecologists for her concern.

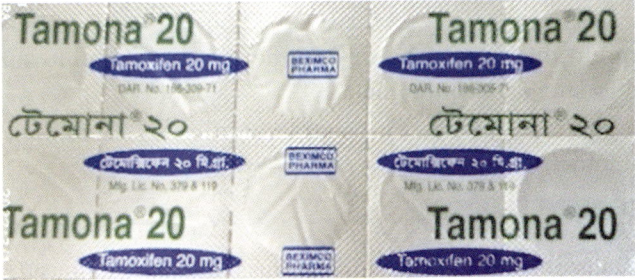

Fig. 11: Tablet tamoxifen.

Endometrial Carcinoma

21.1. Enlist three important information about which the lady should be counseled. (1 × 3 = 3)

21.2. How does tamoxifen induce endometrial cancer? (1 × 2 = 2)

Answer 21.1

1. The patient should use contraception to avoid conception because tamoxifen is teratogenic.
2. She should report immediately to hospital if she notices abnormal vaginal bleeding, spotting, or discharge for prompt assessment by transvaginal ultrasound (TVUS), biopsy, or hysteroscopy and curettage.
3. Tamoxifen use is associated with risk of:
   - Endometrial hyperplasia
   - Endometrial polyp
   - Endometrial cancer
   - Uterine sarcoma
   - Venous thromboembolism (VTE)
   - Stroke

The risk of EC is 2–3-fold increased in these patients than the general population.

Answer 21.2

Tamoxifen acts as an anti-estrogen in breast but exerts estrogenic effect on uterus at standard dose. This unopposed estrogen on the uterus causes endometrial hyperplasia. Subsequently with time, there is progression of disease causing atypical hyperplasia and endometrial cancer. The risk of EC with tamoxifen is mainly related to duration of use. The risk rises after 2 years of use of tamoxifen.

Question 22

A 52-year-old lady who is on tamoxifen for 2 years developed postmenopausal bleeding. Following completion of treatment for breast cancer, she reported to the gynecologist for evaluation.

22.1. Outline the stepwise action the gynecologist should undertake. (0.5 × 3 = 1.5)

22.2. Should this patient be on routine ultrasonographic surveillance while she was asymptomatic. (1.5)

22.3. Enumerate briefly the characteristics of tamoxifen-induced endometrial cancer. (2)

Answer 22.1

Step 1: Details of history on postmenopausal bleeding followed by vaginal examination according to the protocol should be done.

Step 2: Initial work-up by TVUS or hysteroscopy to determine endometrial thickness and/or endometrial polyp.
Step 3: D&C to exclude atypical hyperplasia and/or endometrial cancer.

Answer 22.2

Routine surveillance by TVUS in asymptomatic women on tamoxifen is not beneficial because of its low specificity and positive predictive value. Moreover, it causes anxiety, botheration, and overtreatment.

Answer 22.3

- Evidence has shown that tamoxifen-induced EC is aggressive in behavior and show poor survival outcome in terms of progression-free survival (PFS) and OS.
- Many studies have shown EC is of type II histology or type I histology with poor prognostic factors such as higher grade, deep myometrial invasion, and pelvic and para-aortic lymph node metastasis.

Question 23

A 32-year-old lady having two daughters had breast cancer which is infiltrating duct cell carcinoma. She underwent mastectomy with axillary clearance followed by radiotherapy and chemotherapy. For the last 1 year, she has been on tamoxifen. The lady wants to conceive again and has consulted with a gynecologist.

23.1. The patient should not be allowed for conception. Justify. (2)
23.2. If the patient becomes pregnant with tamoxifen, what will be your advice? (1.5)
23.3. If the patient strongly desires pregnancy in spite of the counseling, what will be your advice for planning pregnancy? (1.5)

Answer 23.1

For effective preventive strategy, tamoxifen is given for 5–10 years to prevent recurrence. It is ideal for the patient not to try for conception during this time.

Tamoxifen does not cause infertility. Due to longer duration of treatment, pregnancy is delayed as the drug is teratogenic, which indirectly interferes in childbearing.

Answer 23.2

Tamoxifen is considered teratogenic. It causes genitourinary developmental defects. Thus, if pregnancy occurs, termination should be advised by safest means.

Answer 23.3

The patient should stop tamoxifen. She should continue contraception for 2 more months before trying for conception. Tamoxifen has a long half-life. It takes 2 months to be eliminated from the body.

Question 24

A 67-year-old postmenopausal lady was diagnosed as endometrial cancer grade 3. Ultrasonography (USG) revealed a complex adnexal mass 6 × 8 cm. She went to gynecologic oncologist for further management.

24.1. What are the correlations of adnexal mass with endometrial cancer? (0.5 × 2 = 1)
24.2. Enumerate the prognosis of patient if there is synchronous primary cancer of the endometrium and ovary. (1.5 + 0.5 = 2)
24.3. What is the standard treatment when synchronous primary endometrial and ovarian cancer is encountered? (0.5 + 1.5 = 2)

Answer 24.1

The correlations are:
- Synchronous primary cancer of the endometrium and ovary which occurs in 5% of all women with endometrial cancer
- Endometrial cancer with adnexal metastasis

Answer 24.2

- Synchronous cancer patients usually are seen to have:
  - Early stage
  - Favorable histologic type
  - Unilateral mass
  - Small endometrial lesions with superficial invasion to endometrium
- These patients have overall good prognosis with 5-year survival of 85% which is better than those with metastatic endometrial cancer.

Answer 24.3

- The standard surgery involves hysterectomy and BSO with or without removal of pelvic lymph node.
- Completion surgery on ovarian protocol should be done which consists of infracolic omentectomy, peritoneal biopsies, and washings. Pelvic lymph node dissection (PLND) as a part of FIGO staging is performed.

Endometrial Carcinoma

Question 25

A 44-year-old lady reported with the diagnosis of endometrial cancer. On preoperative evaluation, the diagnosis was inconclusive. So, decision for intraoperative evaluation by frozen section was taken.

25.1. What is the role of the frozen section in the intraoperative evaluation of endometrial cancer? (2)

25.2. How reliable is frozen section in characterizing risk factors of endometrial cancer? (3)

Answer 25.1

The role of frozen section in the intraoperative evaluation of endometrial cancer is diminishing nowadays because of existence of standard preoperative evaluation system using:
- Curettage specimen
- Imaging studies such as USG, MRI, and computed tomography (CT)
- SLN mapping which accurately predicts lymph node metastasis.

Answer 25.2

When frozen section is compared with final pathology, it shows:
- Highest concordance rate for:
  - Endometrioid histology
  - Myometrial invasion
  - Cervical stromal involvement
- The discordance is for non-endometrioid histology.
- The accuracy for grading tumor ranges between 30 and 60% and disagreement is mostly seen in grade 1 and grade 2 tumors.
- The accuracy for determining lymph node metastasis is 75%.

Question 26

An elderly obese woman reported with postmenopausal bleeding. MRI revealed growth involving both endometrium and cervix. Endometrial and endocervical sampling revealed adenocarcinoma. Considering the age and obesity, diagnosis of endometrial adenocarcinoma was established.

26.1. What is the stage of the disease? Enumerate the standard current approach of treatment for the stage. (0.5 + 2.5 = 3)

26.2. What will be the adjuvant treatment? (1)

26.3. How will you differentiate stage IB adenocarcinoma of cervix from this stage? (1)

Endometrial Carcinoma

Answer 26.1

- The disease is endometrial adenocarcinoma stage II.
- The standard current approach is:
  - Modified radical hysterectomy
  - BSO
  - Peritoneal washing
  - Pelvic lymphadenectomy
  - Resection of enlarged para-aortic nodes
  - Omental biopsy

Answer 26.2

Adjuvant treatment is individualized.
- If lymph nodes are negative, no adjuvant radiation is needed.
- Patients with nodal metastasis should receive either EBRT or extended field external beam radiation.

Answer 26.3

Differentiation is done by IHC staining for P16, which is a surrogate marker for human papillomavirus (HPV) virus and is positive in stage IB adenocarcinoma of cervix. Thus, if P16 is negative in IHC, it indicates EC.

CHAPTER 5

Gestational Trophoblastic Neoplasia

Question 1

A young recently married lady was diagnosed with gestational trophoblastic neoplasia (GTN) following complete molar pregnancy. She reported to the hospital for management.

1.1. What is the prevalence of progression of molar subtypes to GTN? (0.5)
1.2. Outline briefly the workup of GTN apart from clinical evaluation. Justify the need of each workup. (0.5 × 6 = 3)
1.3. Patients of complete hydatidiform mole (CHM) are categorized as high risk or low risk, based on their risk of developing postmolar GTN. Which patients are categorized as high risk? Mention three high risk factors. (0.5 × 3 = 1.5)

Answer 1.1

- CHM progresses to GTN in 15–20% cases.
- Partial hydatidiform mole (PHM) progresses only in 0.5–5% patients to GTN.

Answer 1.2

Work-up of GTN
- *Laboratory studies:*
  - Serum beta-human chorionic gonadotropin (β-hCG) to evaluate tumor burden
  - Complete blood count (CBC), blood grouping, and Rh-typing—to determine the hematological status
  - Renal function test and liver function test—to assess normality in anticipation of future chemotherapy
- *Imaging studies:*
  - Ultrasonogram of pelvis—to determine the extent of tumor
  - Chest X-ray and if needed, chest computed tomography (CT)—to evaluate tumor burden

Answer 1.3

Those patients are classified as high risk who show evidence of marked trophoblastic proliferation such as:
1. Markedly elevated hCG level >100,000 mIU/mL
2. Excessive enlargement of uterus
3. Bilateral theca luteal cysts

Question 2

A woman who is diagnosed as molar pregnancy underwent suction evacuation. Postsuction histopathology revealed CHM **(Fig. 1)**.

   2.1. Enlist three important histological findings that suggest complete hydatidiform mole (CHM).   (0.25 × 3 = 0.75)

   2.2. Differentiate CHM from PHM based on cytogenetics. How the diagnosis of CHM can be confirmed?   (1.25 + 1 = 2.25)

   2.3. Outline the post-treatment surveillance of molar pregnancy.   (1 + 1 = 2)

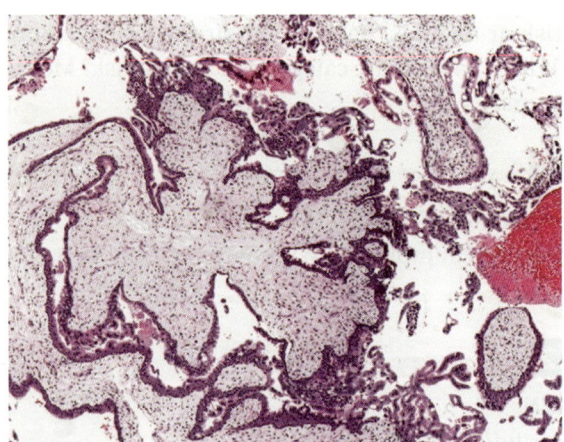

Fig. 1: Complete hydatidiform mole (microscopic).

Answer 2.1

Important histological findings suggestive of CHM are:
1. Trophoblastic proliferation
2. Absence of fetal parts
3. Significant cytological atypia and mitotic figure in villous stroma

Answer 2.2

- CHM is diploid and has 46XX chromosomes with both XX from paternal origin, whereas PHM is triploid and has 69XXY chromosomes with maternal and paternal genetic origin.

- CHM can be confirmed by immune histochemistry (IHC). In CHM, IHC does not show any P57 nuclear staining which is strong in PHM.

Answer 2.3

Following treatment, weekly serum β-hCG should be done till the serum β-hCG is normalized.

For PHM, a single additional normal hCG measurement 1 month after hCG normalization is recommended.

For CHM, monthly hCG measurement should be obtained for 6 months after hCG normalization.

Question 3

A 27-year-old lady underwent a suction evacuation for molar pregnancy. 6 weeks after evacuation, she started having vaginal bleeding and there was rise of hCG in 3 consecutive weekly measurements. Chest X-ray and ultrasonography (USG) of pelvis revealed normal lung and genital organs.

3.1. What is the diagnosis? Mention the stage of the disease.
$(0.5 + 0.5 = 1)$

3.2. If the serum β-hCG is 132,560 mIU/mL, what is the World Health Organization (WHO) prognostic score and risk category of the patient? $(0.5 \times 2 = 1)$

3.3. Enumerate in details the recommended treatment in this patient. What is the anticipated response? $(1 + 0.5 \times 2 + 1 = 3)$

Answer 3.1

The diagnosis is GTN, the International Federation of Gynaecology and Obstetrics (FIGO) stage I.

Answer 3.2

World Health Organization prognostic score is 4.
The risk category is low-risk GTN.

Answer 3.3

- The recommended treatment for low-risk GTN is single agent methotrexate (MTX) 50 mg **(Fig. 2)** intramuscularly on an 8-day regimen.
- Injection MTX is given on days 1, 3, 5, and 7 with 15 mg of folinic acid (FA) on days 2, 4, 6, and 8. The same regimen is repeated every 2 weeks till serum β-hCG returns to normal. Additional one course of injection MTX is given after normalization of serum β-hCG.
- Since the patient is nonmetastatic and in low-risk category, the response to single-agent chemotherapy is excellent. The remission rate is 100% with minimum toxicity.

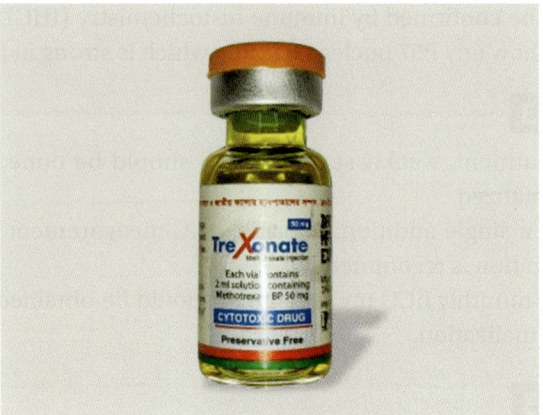

Fig. 2: Injection methotrexate.

Question 4

A 30-year-old woman attended the outpatient department with complain of amenorrhea for 4 months with cough, hemoptysis, and dyspnea for the last 1 month. Transvaginal sonography (TVS) revealed an enlarged uterus with multiple vesicular structures suggesting molar pregnancy. Chest X-ray showed a snowstorm pattern of opacities **(Fig. 3)**. Serum β-hCG was 440,600 mIU/mL.

4.1. What is the diagnosis? (1)

4.2. What is the recommended first-line treatment? Outline the importance of WHO prognostic score. (0.5 × 3 + 1 = 2.5)

4.3. If the patient fails to achieve complete remission and develops resistance (a) to above treatment (b) to both single agents, what action should be taken? (1.5)

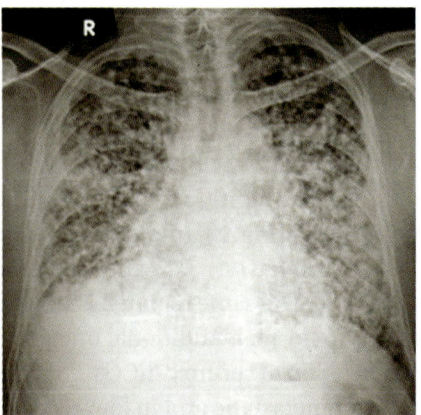

Fig. 3: Snowstorm appearance in chest X-ray.

Answer 4.1
GTN stage III, low-risk group (score 4)

Answer 4.2
- The recommended first-line treatment is single-agent injection MTX with alternate FA.
- WHO prognostic score:
  - Assist in selecting appropriate chemotherapy
  - Determines the likelihood of drug resistance
  - Determines prognosis of disease

Answer 4.3
- If patient develops drug resistance to above treatment, injection MTX-FA is switched to injection actinomycin D **(Fig. 4)**.
- If patient develops drug resistance to both single agents, combination chemotherapy should be started.

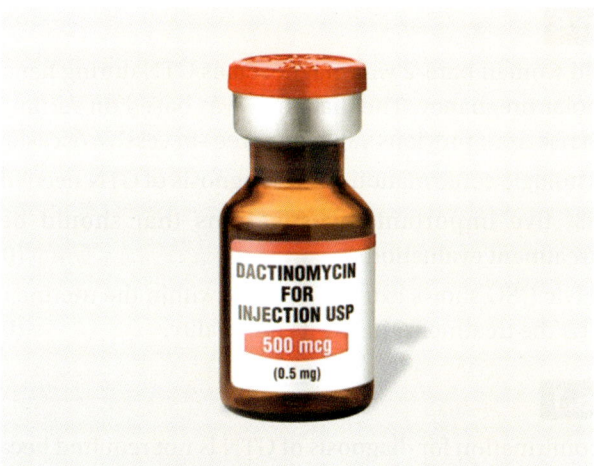

Fig. 4: Injection actinomycin D.

Question 5
A young woman has been treated with single-agent chemotherapy for nonmetastatic GTN. She is now on follow-up.
- 5.1. Enumerate the schedule of follow-up of this patient. (1 + 1 = 2)
- 5.2. What is the risk of relapse in such a patient? (1)
- 5.3. Which contraception is advised and why it is essential during follow-up? (1 + 1 = 2)

Answer 5.1

The schedule of follow-up is:
- Weekly measurement of hCG until they are normal for three consecutive weeks.
- Monthly hCG levels until they are normal for 12 consecutive months.

Answer 5.2

The risk of relapse is <5% in the first year following completion of treatment. Thereafter, the relapse is extremely low.

Answer 5.3

Barrier method and oral contraceptive—anyone can be advised but oral contraceptives are definitely effective.

Contraception is essential because if the patient becomes pregnant during follow-up, it will create confusion whether the rise in serum hCG is due to pregnancy or relapse.

Question 6

A 35-year-old woman para-2 was diagnosed as GTN during her surveillance following molar pregnancy. The diagnosis was based on serum hCG which showed 10% rise from previous value on three successive occasions.

6.1. Is histologic confirmation of the diagnosis of GTN needed? (1)

6.2. Enlist five important investigations that should be done for pretreatment evaluation. (0.5 × 5 = 2.5)

6.3. If pelvic USG shows extensive tumor within the uterine cavity, what will be the treatment? Justify its rationality. (0.5 + 1 = 1.5)

Answer 6.1

Histologic confirmation for diagnosis of GTN is not required because in only one-third patients, histological evidence of GTN can be found as evident in literature.

The diagnosis is established mostly on the basis of clinical and biological parameters.

Answer 6.2

For pretreatment evaluation, following investigation should be done:
- Serum hCG
- Chest X-ray, if positive chest CT
- Blood for CBC, hepatic, thyroid, and renal function tests
- Pelvic ultrasound

Gestational Trophoblastic Neoplasia

Answer 6.3

Hysterectomy **(Fig. 5)** can be the treatment of choice and is favorable in the above scenario.

It will reduce tumor burden and limit the number of cycles of chemotherapy necessary to induce remission. Moreover, hysterectomy will eliminate the possibilities for hemorrhage and infection.

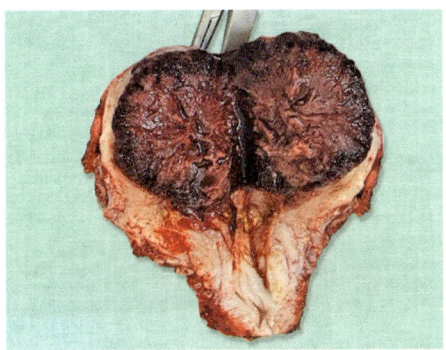

Fig. 5: Hysterectomy specimen with gestational trophoblastic neoplasia (GTN).

Question 7

A 28-year-old lady was diagnosed as GTN 8 months following suction evacuation for molar pregnancy. At diagnosis, she had a serum β-hCG of 365,489 mIU/mL and multiple cannon ball rounded opacities in both lungs **(Fig. 6)**.

7.1. How will you stratify the patient? Demonstrate risk factors according to WHO prognostic score. $(0.5 \times 6 = 3)$

7.2. Which regimen of chemotherapy will be used in this patient and what will be the outcome? $(1.5 + 0.5 = 2)$

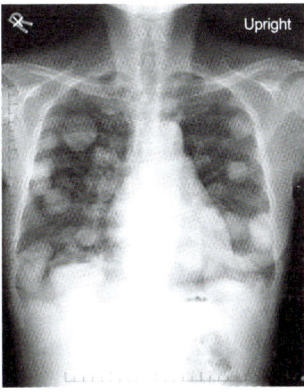

Fig. 6: Cannon ball opacities in both lungs.

Answer 7.1

Stratification of the patient will be done according to WHO prognostic factor.

   WHO prognostic score = 7
   The patient belongs to the high-risk category.

TABLE 1: World Health Organization (WHO) prognostic score according to scenario.

	0	1	2	4
Age	√			
Antecedent pregnancy	√			
Interval from index pregnancy			√	
Pretreatment serum β-hCG				√
Site of metastasis		Lung		
Number of metastasis		√		

(β-hCG: beta-human chorionic gonadotropin)

Answer 7.2

Combination chemotherapy: EMACO regimen is commonly used.

EMACO consists of etoposide, methotrexate, actinomycin-D, cyclophosphamide, and oncovin/vincristine, which is repeated every 2 weeks.

The outcome is good with a complete response rate in 80–90% of patients.

Question 8

A patient developed high-risk GTN during follow-up following spontaneous abortion. She was prescribed EMACO chemotherapy after systematic evaluation.

   8.1. What is the duration of chemotherapy? (1.5)
   8.2. What are the expected toxicities in such combination therapy? (1.5)
   8.3. If during treatment, patient shows plateau of serum β-hCG for 3 successive weeks, what does it indicate? What remedy should be undertaken? (0.5 + 1.5 = 2)

Answer 8.1

The EMACO chemotherapy **(Fig. 7)** is given until normal hCG is achieved.

After normal β-hCG level, two additional courses of chemotherapy are given as consolidation therapy to reduce the risk of relapse.

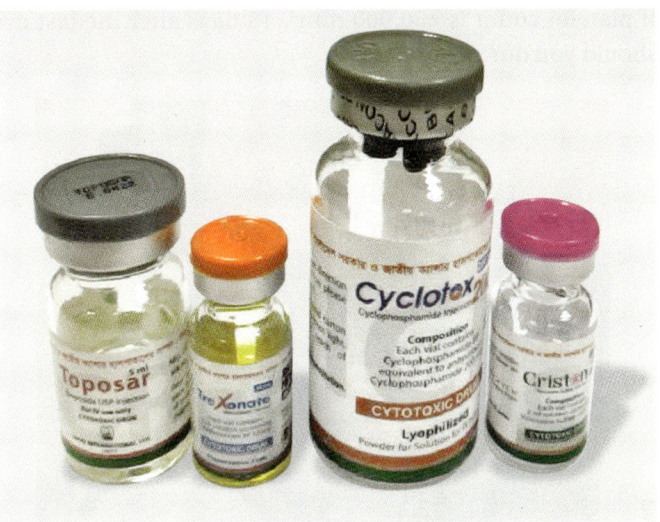

Fig. 7: Drugs included in EMACO therapy.

Answer 8.2

There is 1.5-fold risk of developing secondary tumors 10–25 years after therapy particularly if etoposide is used.

The secondary tumors include myeloid leukemia, colon cancer, melanoma, and breast cancer.

Answer 8.3

It indicates drug resistance.

Remedy:
- Modification of EMACO regimen by substituting etoposide and cisplatin (EP) on day 8 for cyclophosphamide and vincristine. Then, the regimen will be EMA-EP (etoposide methotrexate and actinomycin-D/EP).
- Surgical intervention can be done to remove resistant tumors based on individual's reproductive background.

Question 9

A woman is undergoing treatment for high-risk GTN by EMACO **(Fig. 8)**. She is on regular monitoring during treatment.

    9.1. Why is monitoring essential in between treatments? How will you monitor her between treatment? (1 + 1.5 = 2.5)

    9.2. What parameter will indicate that the response of treatment is satisfactory? (1.5)

9.3. If platelet count is <50,000 mm³, 13 days after the last cycle, what should you do? (1)

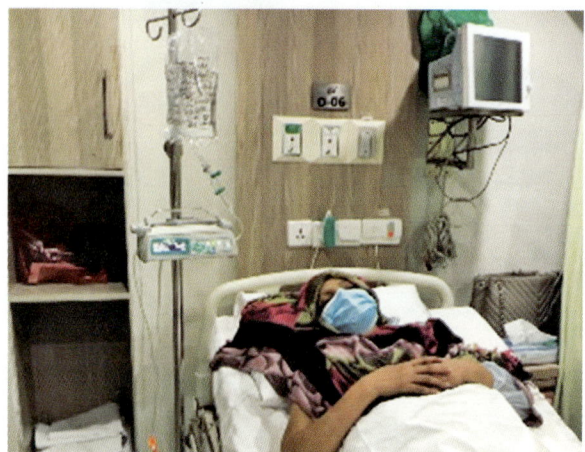

Fig. 8: Patient receiving chemotherapy in day care unit.

Answer 9.1

- Monitoring during chemotherapy is essential to:
    - Evaluate the response of treatment.
    - Evaluate toxicity.
- Monitoring is done in between courses of treatment by:
    - History
    - Physical examination
    - Biochemical tests
- Detail history on:
    - Gastrointestinal tract (GIT) symptoms
    - Stomatitis
    - Alopecia
    - Skin rash
- Physical examination:
    - Exclude vaginal metastasis
- Biochemical tests include:
    - Serum β-hCG
    - CBC
    - Renal function tests
    - Liver function tests

Answer 9.2

Response of treatment is evaluated by serum β-hCG in between courses of treatment.

If the fall of serum β-hCG is >10% of previous week titer, it is satisfactory and further chemotherapy is continued as per schedule.

Answer 9.3

It indicates toxicity and thus treatment should be withheld.

Fresh blood should be given to raise platelet concentration. Once platelet level reaches to normal, then treatment should be started.

Question 10

A young lady who has been treated by EMACO therapy for high-risk GTN is now under post-treatment surveillance. She wants to become pregnant and has come for suggestions.

10.1. When should the lady be allowed to become pregnant? Give explanation. (1 + 1.5 = 2.5)
10.2. What special precautions should be undertaken when the patient becomes pregnant and following delivery? (0.5 × 3 = 1.5)
10.3. How long does this patient need to be followed up? (1)

Answer 10.1

The lady should avoid pregnancy for 1½ years following completion of treatment.

The chemotherapy has teratogenic effect on mature ova which are spontaneously eliminated from the body during 1 year following completion of treatment. The resting oocytes are not affected by chemotherapy. Thus, after 1½ year, the patient can try for pregnancy when there will be no risk of teratogenicity.

Answer 10.2

If the patient becomes pregnant:
- USG should be done in the first trimester to confirm normal gestational development.
- Placenta should be sent for histopathology after delivery to confirm normal placental tissue.
- Serum β-hCG should be estimated 6 weeks after delivery to exclude occult trophoblastic disease.

Answer 10.3

The patient needs to be followed up for 5 years after completion of treatment. The patient will be declared cured if she remains asymptomatic and serum β-hCG is normal.

104   Gestational Trophoblastic Neoplasia

Question 11

A woman had irregular on and off bleeding for 1 year following full-term pregnancy. She was treated by local doctors with progesterone but was not improved. In the meantime, she developed headache, vertigo, and blurring of vision. Magnetic resonance imaging (MRI) revealed brain metastasis **(Fig. 9)**. Subsequently, the woman was diagnosed as GTN.

11.1. What is the stage and risk category of disease? (1)
11.2. What is the standard treatment? (1.5)
11.3. What is the role of craniotomy? Outline the prognosis of the disease. (1.5 + 1 = 2.5)

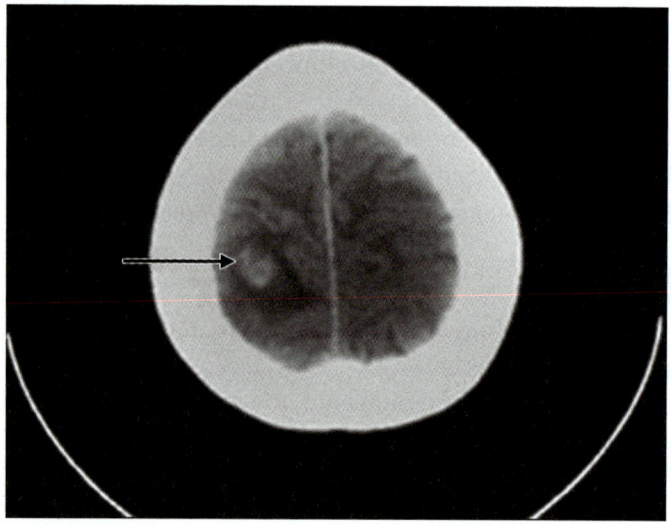

Fig. 9: Magnetic resonance imaging (MRI) showing brain metastasis in GTN.

Answer 11.1

Stage IV, high-risk GTN.

Answer 11.2

- EP-EMA is the preferred regimen here with four cycles of consolidation chemotherapy.
- 3,000 CGy whole brain irradiation is given with concurrent chemotherapy. Here, brain irradiation is both hemostatic and tumoricidal.

Answer 11.3

- Craniotomy in brain metastasis is indicated:
  - When acute decompression is needed in hemorrhage.

- When cerebral metastases are resistant to chemotherapy, particularly if located peripherally.
■ GTN with cerebral metastases is associated with very poor prognosis. Early or late death is associated with brain hemorrhage or resistant to treatment, respectively.

Question 12

A 45-year-old woman after treatment of complete mole, during surveillance presented with huge abdominal distention and hypovolemic shock. Her preoperative β-hCG level was 455,640 mIU/mL. Chest X-ray and other imaging studies did not reveal any metastasis. After laparotomy, an enlarged uterus containing molar tissue perforating through the uterine wall was seen.

12.1. What is the diagnosis? (1)
12.2. Which histological finding confirms the diagnosis? (1.5)
12.3. What is the standard treatment in this case? What is the role of chemotherapy here? (1 + 1.5 = 2.5)

Answer 12.1

The diagnosis is invasive mole which is a subtype of GTN that develops from malignant transformation of trophoblastic tissue after molar evacuation.

Answer 12.2

Chorionic villi invading the myometrium with or without uterine vessels invasion which is surrounded by proliferating trophoblastic cells **(Fig. 10)** in specimen of uterus histologically confirms the diagnosis.

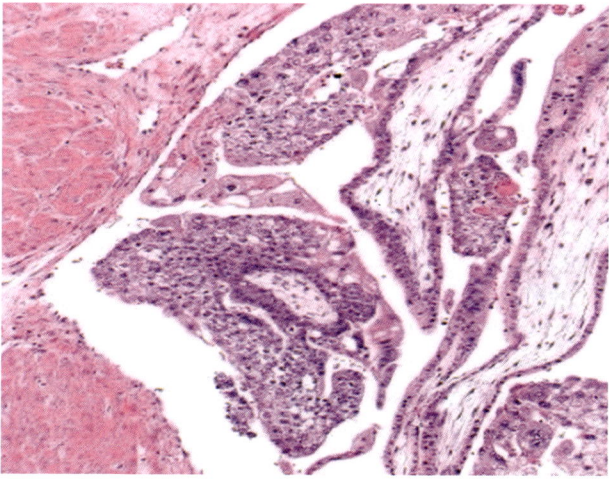

Fig. 10: Histological diagnosis of invasive mole.

Answer 12.3

- As there is perforation of the uterus with uncontrolled intraperitoneal bleeding resulting in shock, immediate surgery is needed. The standard recommended treatment is total abdominal hysterectomy.
- Invasive moles are highly sensitive to chemotherapy and are considered first-line treatment in most of the cases. Postoperative single-agent chemotherapy is given to prevent activation of occult metastases.

Question 13

A woman was diagnosed as ultra-high risk GTN, 3 years after full-term pregnancy. She had liver and brain metastasis and FIGO scoring was >12.

13.1. The standard treatment is multiagent chemotherapy? What is the risk involved when such aggressive treatment is started at onset? (1.5)

13.2. Which strategies are helpful to avoid the problems? (0.5 × 4 = 2)

13.3. What are the different chemotherapy regimen used in such situation? (1.5)

Answer 13.1

Once multiagent chemotherapy is started, the patient is at risk of:
- Bleeding or intratumoral hemorrhage into metastatic sites
- Organ failure

This happens due to rapid tumor collapse or tumor lysis syndrome once chemotherapy is started.

Answer 13.2

- Starting chemotherapy slowly (low-dose induction of etoposide)
- Ensuring adequate hydration
- Close monitoring of electrolyte and renal function
- Preferably treating patients in high-dependency or intensive care units

Answer 13.3

- The first-line regimen is EP/EMA in alternating weeks or EP + intrathecal MTX/EMA (CNS).
- If there is ascites, there is pooling of MTX, the treatment of choice is paclitaxel and cisplatin alternating every 2 weeks with paclitaxel and etoposide.

Question 14

A patient is on surveillance following treatment for high-risk GTN. On 9th month during follow-up, she came to the outdoor with the complaint of nausea, vomiting, headache, and blurring of vision.

14.1. Which investigation will be preferred in such situation? (1)

14.2. If MRI of the brain is negative but the symptoms persist what action should be taken? Outline the findings in cerebrospinal fluid (CSF) if brain metastasis is present. (2 + 1 = 3)

14.3. How long should the patient be followed up following completion of treatment? (1)

Answer 14.1

Magnetic resonance imaging of the brain.

Answer 14.2

- Baseline investigations should be done which includes:
  - CBC
  - Serum β-hCG
  - Liver function test
  - Renal function test
  - Chest X-ray
  - hCG in CSF
- The plasma/CSF hCG ratio is <60.

Answer 14.3

Since the patient had recurrence within 1 year of follow-up, she should be kept under close monitoring for lifelong.

Question 15

A 40-year-old woman underwent suction evacuation for molar pregnancy. Histologically, the molar tissue revealed intermediate trophoblastic cells, sheets of anaplastic syncytiotrophoblasts, and cytotrophoblasts in absence of chorionic villi **(Fig. 11)**.

15.1. What is the diagnosis? Name four antecedent pregnancies which depict choriocarcinoma. (1 + 0.25 × 4 = 2)

15.2. Which immunohistochemistry parameters can confirm the diagnosis? (1.5)

15.3. After two cycles of single-agent chemotherapy, serum β-hCG was raised >10% of previous week in consecutive 3 weeks. What should be done now? (1.5)

Answer 15.1

The diagnosis is choriocarcinoma.

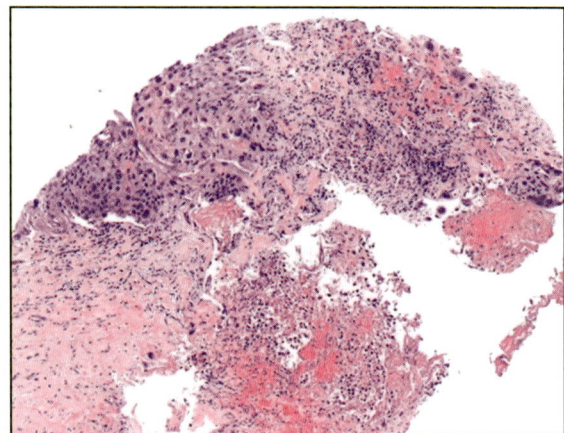

Fig. 11: Microscopic view of choriocarcinoma.

Four antecedent pregnancy which can progress to choriocarcinoma includes:
1. Molar pregnancy
2. Full-term pregnancy
3. Abortion
4. Ectopic pregnancy

Answer 15.2

Immune histochemistry shows:
- β-hCG in syncytiotrophoblast cells—strongly positive
- Ki–67—positive in tumor cells >90%
- Cytokeratin—low in tumor cells

Answer 15.3

Here, the diagnosis is drug resistance.

Since the patient is 40 years, hysterectomy will remove the chemotherapy-resistant tissue in the uterus and thus improve the response to chemotherapy.

Question 16

A 32-year-old lady complained of metrorrhagia for 1 year, 3 years after term pregnancy. The pelvic USG showed no distinctive characteristics.

Serum β-hCG was 560 mIU/mL. Histology following dilation and curettage (D&C) revealed several trophoblastic viable cells with extensive tumor necrosis. The patient was treated with oral contraceptives with monthly follow-up of β-hCG which remained static. IHC was done to confirm the diagnosis.

16.1. What is the probable diagnosis? What parameters in IHC will confirm the diagnosis. (0.5 + 1 = 1.5)

16.2. Mention four factors which will differentiate between the above diagnosis and GTN. (0.5 × 4 = 2)

16.3. If MRI of pelvis reveals the tumor within the uterus but myometrial invasion is >50%, what will be the standard treatment? Outline the prognosis based on scenario. (1 + 0.5 = 1.5)

Answer 16.1

The probable diagnosis is placental site trophoblastic tumor (PSTT).

In human placental lactogen (IHC), tumor cells show:
- Positive staining for HPL
- Negative or partially positive staining for β-hCG
- Negative staining for P63

Answer 16.2

- It is a slowly growing tumor, which tends to remain confined within uterus, metastasizing late in their course.
- It arises from intermediate trophoblast, thus β-hCG levels are low relative to the mass, unlike other GTN.
- They spread through lymphatics while GTN has hematogenous spread.
- They are relatively resistant to chemotherapy in contrast to other GTN.

Answer 16.3

- The standard treatment is total abdominal hysterectomy with pelvic lymph node sampling and conservation of both ovaries.
- The prognosis of the disease is poor. Because:
  - Long interval of 36 months between antecedent pregnancy and development of PSTT
  - Deep myometrial invasion of >50%

Question 17

A 40-year-old woman was diagnosed as GTN, 3½ years after full-term pregnancy. On evaluation, she was found to have multiple metastasis in the liver and the brain. Her serum β-hCG was 567,435 mIU/mL and the prognostic score was 14.

17.1. What is the GTN subtype in the scenario? Specify the extent of tumor burden here. (1 + 0.5 × 3 = 2.5)
17.2. Outline the treatment protocol. (0.5 × 3 = 1.5)
17.4. What will be the response to chemotherapy in this case? (1)

Answer 17.1

Ultra-high risk GTN

The woman had high tumor burden as evident by:
- Multiple metastasis in the liver and the brain
- High serum β-hCG of 567,435 mIU/mL
- High WHO prognostic score-14

Answer 17.2

- Low-dose induction chemotherapy with EP weekly for 3 weeks until patient's condition is improved.
- Standard chemotherapy protocol of EMA is commenced thereafter and continued until β-hCG is normalized.
- Additional four cycles of consolidation therapy is given.

Answer 17.3

The response to chemotherapy is variable.

Use of low-dose induction chemotherapy with intensive specialist support has shown good outcomes but significant number of patients will develop drug resistance and will die from the disease.

Question 18

A 28-year-old nulliparous lady is diagnosed as stage III GTN with prognostic score 9.

18.1. What is the preferred primary treatment in this case? Give reasons. (0.5 + 0.5 × 3 = 2)
18.2. If the patient is resistant to above treatment, what is the alternative regime? (1.5)
18.3. When etoposide is used, why it is important to counsel the patient and family pretreatment? (1.5)

Answer 18.1

Combination chemotherapy EMACO regimen is the preferred.

Reasons for preference:
- The patient is in stage III which means tumor has spread to the lung with or without spread to ovary, fallopian tube, vagina, and/or connective tissue around the uterus.
- WHO prognostic score is high.
- The response rate is excellent with minimum toxicity and is well tolerated.

Answer 18.2

If the patient is resistant to EMACO, the alternate regimen is EMA-EP, where cyclophosphamide and vincristine are replaced by EP.

Evidence has shown a response rate of 65–75% with EMA-EP in patient who are resistant to EMACO.

Answer 18.3

With etoposide **(Fig. 12)** use, there is risk of developing secondary tumors such as acute myeloid leukemia, melanoma, colon cancer, and breast cancer. Thus, the patient must be informed about this before treatment.

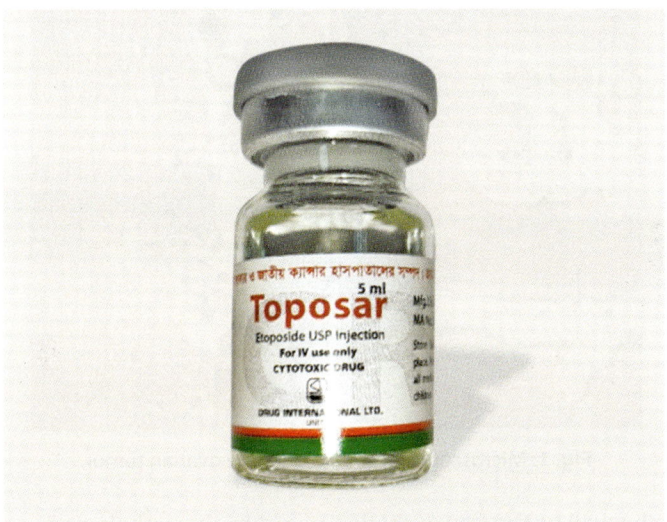

Fig. 12: Vial-containing injection etoposide.

CHAPTER 6

Epithelial Ovarian Cancer

Question 1

A 32-year-old lady, para-1 presents with an adnexal mass of 8 × 6 cm. Intraoperatively the mass was in one ovary which was encapsulated. There was no evidence of metastasis in other organs within the abdominal cavity. Frozen section analysis during surgery revealed high cellular proliferation, nuclear atypia, mitotic activity, papillary structure formation but no stromal invasion **(Fig. 1)**.

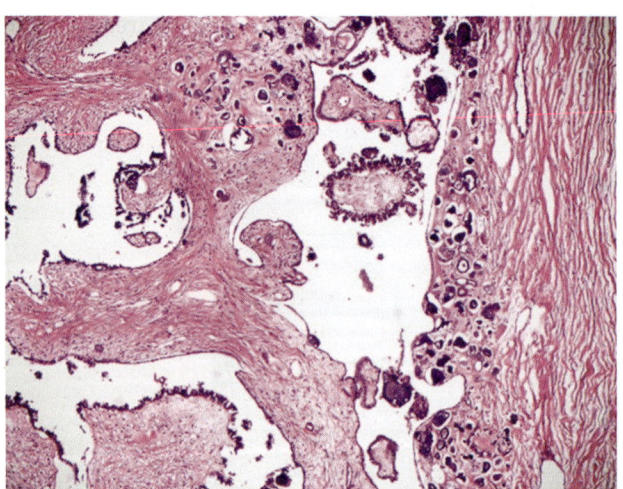

Fig. 1: Microscopic view of borderline ovarian tumor.

1.1. What will be the frozen section report by the pathologist? (1)
1.2. If the patient desires fertility preservation, discuss the surgical option that should be offered. Explain in which condition fertility sparing surgery should not be done. (1.5 + 1 = 2.5)
1.3. If it is an advanced stage disease, explain the role of adjuvant treatment. (1.5)

Answer 1.1

Borderline ovarian tumor (BOT).

Answer 1.2

- Unilateral salpingo-oophorectomy of the involved ovary with surgical staging which includes peritoneal cytology, exploration, omentectomy, and multiple peritoneal biopsies. Lymphadenectomy without bulky lymph nodes is not indicated.
- Completion of standard surgical procedure, i.e., hysterectomy and salpingo-oophorectomy of remaining ovary is recommended when family is complete.

If the histologic type of BOT is endometrioid, fertility sparing surgery cannot be done even if the patient desires because the uterus remains at risk of subsequent endometrial cancer.

Answer 1.3

- The available data do not confirm the efficacy of adjuvant therapy (chemotherapy or radiotherapy) in advanced stage of BOT in the improvement of prognosis rather it causes significant toxicities.
- In recurrent BOT, same concept exists. Thus, the treatment of choice in all BOT is surgery aiming at complete tumor resection.

Question 2

A 38-year-old woman reported with an advanced stage ovarian tumor. Frozen section reported a diagnosis of serous borderline tumor (SBT). The lady underwent total abdominal hysterectomy with bilateral salpingo-oophorectomy.

    2.1. How reliable is the frozen section in the diagnosis of BOT? (1.5)
    2.2. What is the role of relaparotomy in this case? (2)
    2.3. How will this patient be followed up? Why it is essential to follow-up the patient? (1.5)

Answer 2.1

The accuracy of the frozen section in the diagnosis of BOT is low. 20–30% of ovarian tumors diagnosed as borderline at frozen section may prove to be invasive carcinoma on final histopathology. This discordance is more specifically seen in mucinous tumors.

Answer 2.2

- The role of the relaparotomy for completion of surgery in BOT is controversial. Omentectomy and pelvic lymphadenectomy if not done in primary surgery in BOT do not affect the survival of the patient.

- ROBOT study has reported incomplete staging as independent risk factor for recurrence, but there is no therapeutic implication because lymph node does not affect prognosis. If repeat surgery is done when recurrence is diagnosed, there is prolonged survival which is equivalent to survival achieved at relaparotomy. Thus, there is no need of relaparotomy in this case.

Answer 2.3

- The patient will be followed up by history, physical examination, abdominopelvic computed tomography (CT) scan, and serum CA-125 level periodically.
- The follow-up is essential to detect recurrence early so that definite surgery can be done.

Question 3

A 32-year-old lady was found to have stage I BOT on frozen section. So conservative surgery in the form of unilateral salpingo-oophorectomy was done **(Fig. 2)**. But the final histology revealed invasive implants within the borderline tumor.

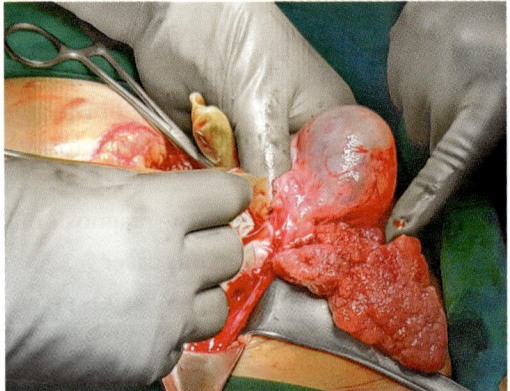

Fig. 2: Intraoperative view of borderline ovarian tumor.

3.1. How should this patient be dealt now? (1.25 + 1.25 = 2.5)
3.2. Explain the role of adjuvant chemotherapy here. (1.25)
3.3. What will be the consequences if such a patient is left untreated? (1.25)

Answer 3.1

- If conservative surgery is done because of fertility issue, the patient should be counseled for quick completion of family and monitoring by

transvaginal sonography (TVS) periodically in the meantime. Once the family is complete, total hysterectomy with removal of another ovary should be done.
- If family is complete, relaparotomy followed by total abdominal hysterectomy with unilateral salpingo-oophorectomy should be done to reduce the risk of recurrence.

Answer 3.2

Adjuvant chemotherapy does not provide any benefit as the borderline tumors have low response to platinum-based chemotherapy because the cells proliferate slowly.

Answer 3.3

There is probability of recurrence of disease or progression to carcinoma but evidence have shown secondary cytoreductive surgery results in satisfactory survival which is equivalent to the survival achieved with relaparotomy.

Question 4

A 47-year-old lady was diagnosed with an early-stage ovarian cancer. The patient was prepared for surgery. At surgery, optimum cytoreduction was achieved, but the oncosurgeon was confused whether to do systematic lymph node dissection or lymph node sampling.

4.1. Compare the reliability of imaging and intraoperative palpation of lymph node beds in detecting lymph node metastasis? (2)

4.2. What is the role of para-aortic and pelvic lymphadenectomy in this case? (1.5)

4.3. Justify which type of lymphadenectomy (systematic or sampling) should be done here. (1.5)

Answer 4.1

- Both imaging [CT scan/magnetic resonance imaging (MRI)] and intraoperative palpation of lymph node beds have low sensitivity and specificity for the detection of lymph node metastasis.
- CT scan/MRI or palpatory method can only detect bulky lymph nodes. Bulky lymph nodes are not always metastatic. Nonbulky lymph nodes can be metastatic which will be missed both by imaging and palpation. Also, both cannot differentiate between metastatic and inflammatory bulky lymph nodes.

Answer 4.2

In early stage ovarian cancer, pelvic and para-aortic lymphadenectomy should be done because:
- It assigns complete staging, thus helps in planning treatment.
- It triages the patient and helps in decision-making regarding the need of adjuvant chemotherapy.
- It provides important prognostic information.

Answer 4.3

- Systematic or sampling lymphadenectomy either can be done in this case because:
  - Evidence suggests that there is no difference in progression-free survival (PFS) and overall survival (OS) in patients with early stage epithelial ovarian carcinoma (EOC) between systematic and sampling lymphadenectomy.

Question 5

Lymph node metastasis is a significant prognostic factor for survival in ovarian carcinoma (EOC). A woman with early-stage epithelial ovarian cancer underwent systematic pelvic and para-aortic lymphadenectomy.

5.1. If the lymph nodes were positive, what would be the surgical stage of disease? (1)

5.2. Enlist three risk factors for lymph node metastasis in early stage ovarian cancer. (0.5 × 3 = 1.5)

5.3. How the para-aortic and pelvic lymph node metastasis occurs in ovarian cancer? (1.5 + 1 = 2.5)

Answer 5.1

Stage IIIA1.

Answer 5.2

- Histologic type—serous
- Histologic grade III
- High serum CA-125

Answer 5.3

- Lymph node metastasis occurs via the retroperitoneal lymphatics draining the ovary. The principal lymphatic drainage of the ovary occurs in para-aortic lymph nodes. The dissemination follows the ovarian vein

and lymphatics in the infundibulopelvic ligament to the lymph nodes lining the aorta and vena cava up to the level of renal vessels.
- The lymph channels can also pass laterally through the broad ligament and parametrium to terminate in the pelvic lymph nodes.

Question 6

A 43-year-old nulliparous lady presented with ovarian cancer with ascites. On laparotomy, tumor was limited within one ovary with intact capsule but the tumor was on the ovarian surface **(Fig. 3)**. Patient had ascites. Uterus, fallopian tube, and all other abdominal organs were healthy. Postoperatively the histology was low-grade serous tumor, G2 with malignant cells in ascites.

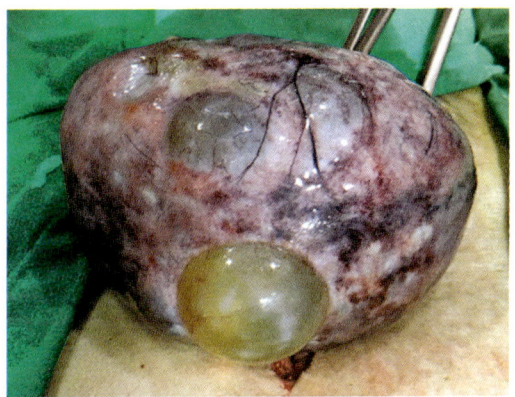

Fig. 3: Serous adenocarcinoma of ovary.

6.1. What is the stage of disease? Enlist three high risk factors in the Disease. (0.75 + 0.25 × 3 = 1.5)
6.2. Outline the primary treatment in such a case. (1 + 0.5 = 1.5)
6.3. Enumerate the steps of pelvic lymph node removal in surgical staging. (1 + 1 = 2)

Answer 6.1

Stage IC3.

High risk factors are:
1. Tumor on surface of ovary
2. Malignant cells in ascitic fluid
3. Ascites

Answer 6.2

Total abdominal hysterectomy with bilateral salpingo-oophorectomy and surgical staging.

Answer 6.3

- Enlarged pelvic lymph node is resected on the ipsilateral side and submitted for frozen section.
- If no metastasis is found, systematic pelvic lymphadenectomy is performed. But if metastasis is found, this step is omitted.

Question 7

A 48-year-old lady presents with ovarian cancer which is bilateral with growth on the surface. There are peritoneal implants <2 cm in size, moderate ascites, and metastatic pelvic lymph nodes **(Fig. 4)**. The histopathology reveals low-grade serous carcinoma (LGSC), grade 2.

7.1. What is the stage of the disease? (0.5)

7.2. Is optimal cytoreduction achievable in this case? Enlist four parameters which will be in favor of surgery. (0.5 + 0.5 × 4 = 2.5)

7.3. What is the prognosis of the disease? Give reasons. (2)

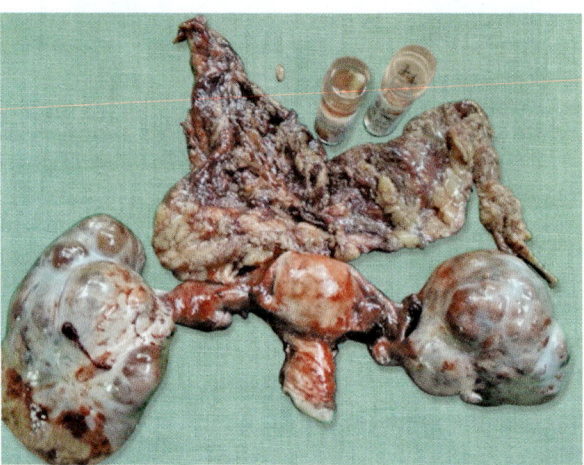

Fig. 4: Structures removed after optimum cytoreduction.

Answer 7.1

The stage is stage IIIB.

Answer 7.2

Optimum cytoreduction is achievable following debulking surgery in this case because:
1. Bilateral ovarian tumors with growth on surface are resectable.
2. Pelvic lymphadenectomy is feasible.

Epithelial Ovarian Cancer 119

3. There is no mesenteric involvement.
4. Peritoneal implants are <2 cm in size.

Answer 7.3

The patient will have an overall good prognosis.
- The patient has LGSC which are indolent in behavior.
- Though the disease is in the advanced stage, optimum cytoreduction is achievable which brings a good outcome.
- The disease is in grade 2.
  Evidence has shown that OS ranges between 5 and 6 years.

Question 8

A postmenopausal woman was diagnosed on laparotomy with epithelial ovarian cancer confined to one ovary with breach of ovarian capsule and ascites **(Fig. 5)**. There was no other evidence of metastasis on exploration. Total abdominal hysterectomy with bilateral salpingo-oophorectomy and surgical staging was done.

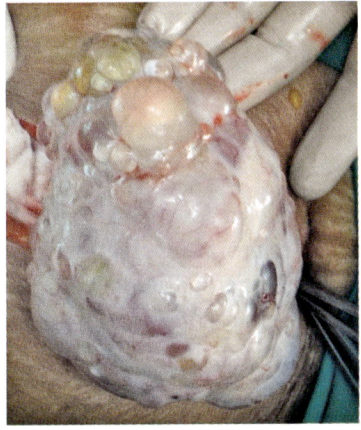

Fig. 5: Ovarian cancer with breach of capsule.

8.1. What is the surgical stage of the disease? Enlist six important information that will be additionally obtained from histopathology and cytology report. (0.5 + 0.5 × 6 = 3.5)
8.2. Justify the need of adjuvant chemotherapy in this case. (1)
8.3. What will be the response to chemotherapy, if histology is LGSC? (0.5)

Answer 8.1

Stage 1C2.

Information that will be obtained after surgery are:
- *From histopathology:*
  1. Histologic subtype
  2. Histologic grade
  3. Size of tumor
  4. Another ovary, fallopian tube, and uterus—metastasis present/absent
  5. Lymphovascular space invasion (LVSI)
  6. Omentum, pelvic lymph nodes, resected site—metastasis present/absent
- *From ascitic fluid cytology:*
  - Malignant cells in ascites present/absent

Answer 8.2

The patient will need adjuvant chemotherapy to prolong PFS and OS. Though it is an early-stage disease, there are high-risk features such as tumor growth on the surface of ovary, ascites which will result in early relapse.

Answer 8.3

- The response rate to chemotherapy is low in LGSC approximately 3–4% because of low proliferating cells.
- There is relapse despite treatment but has relatively longer survival.

Question 9

A 65-year-old lady presented with advanced stage epithelial ovarian cancer. On laparotomy, there was bilateral involvement of both ovaries **(Fig. 6)**, ascites, and dissemination involving the pelvic peritoneum, surface of the bowel and other abdominal organs, uterus, and broad ligament.

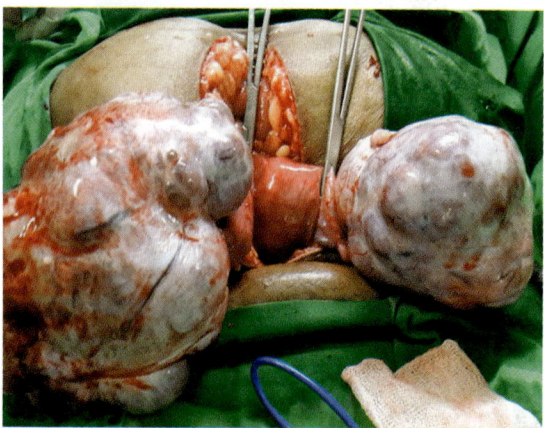

Fig. 6: Advanced stage ovarian cancer with bilateral ovarian involvement.

9.1. How did pelvic and abdominal spread happen? (0.5 × 2 = 1)
9.2. Which two preoperative tumor markers are helpful in diagnosis in this case? (0.5 × 2 = 1)
9.3. Enumerate the information provided by preoperative CT scan to predict optimal cytoreduction here. (3)

Answer 9.1

This is either by:
- Direct extension
- Metastasis when exfoliation of malignant cells results in seedling of peritoneal surfaces

Answer 9.2

Combination of serum CA-125 and HE4 is helpful in diagnosis when raised as they have increased sensitivity and specificity in combination in predicting serous tumors which is responsible for two-thirds of the advanced stage of EOC.

Answer 9.3

Preoperative CT scan can predict the feasibility of optimal cytoreduction by providing the following information:
- CT scan can characterize ovarian tumor and exclude involvement of surrounding organs such as bladder, ureter, sigmoid colon, and pelvic side wall by using contrast (**Fig. 7**).
- CT scan with contrast can identify:
  - Omental and mesenteric involvement
  - Suprarenal and infrarenal lymphadenopathy
  - Large volume ascites
  - Intrahepatic involvement

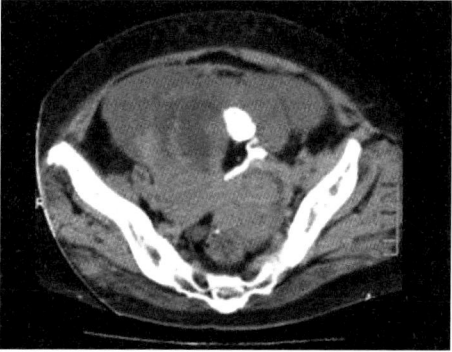

Fig. 7: Computed tomography (CT) scan showing bilateral ovarian involvement in advanced stage epithelial ovarian carcinoma (EOC).

Question 10

A 66-year-old lady with advanced stage epithelial ovarian cancer was scheduled for debulking surgery after thorough preoperative evaluation. The patient was explained in details about the procedure and its benefits.

10.1. What is the goal of debulking surgery? (0.5)

10.2. Enumerate three important benefits of debulking surgery. (1 × 3 = 3)

10.3. Outline the current practice of lymph node removal in advanced stage of EOC. (1.5)

Answer 10.1

- The goal is to resect all visible tumors in the pelvis and abdomen (R_0 stage) in order to achieve optimum cytoreduction.
- If R_0 stage is not achievable, the objective is to resect tumor bulk leaving only 1 cm of residual disease.

Answer 10.2

There are three important benefits:
1. Large, bulky tumors contain necrotic or hypoxic areas that have low growth fraction (large proportion of cells are in the G_0 phase of cell cycle) and are resistant to chemotherapy. Removal of such masses enhances the response of the remaining tumor to chemotherapy.
2. Removal of tumor masses produces significant symptoms relief from tumor externally pressing on organs in the pelvis or upper abdomen.
3. Tumor debulking reduces ascites and enhances the patient's ability to maintain her nutritional and functional status, resulting in higher quality of life.

Answer 10.3

The current practice is to remove enlarged or suspicious lymph nodes as part of tumor debulking because systematic lymphadenectomy improves PFS but not OS.

However, patients where optimum cytoreduction is achievable, systematic pelvic and para-aortic lymph node dissection is done because it might therapeutically benefit the patient.

Question 11

A 62-year-old postmenopausal lady presented with advanced epithelial ovarian cancer. She was selected for primary debulking surgery (PDS). There was a solid mass in the upper abdomen correlating to omental cake **(Fig. 8)**.

11.1. Enlist four other causes of upper abdominal mass. (0.25 × 4 = 1)

11.2. What is the relationship between residual tumor and survival tumor? (1.5)
11.3. Explain the mechanism of feasibility of safely removal of omental cake without any injury to intestine. (2.5)

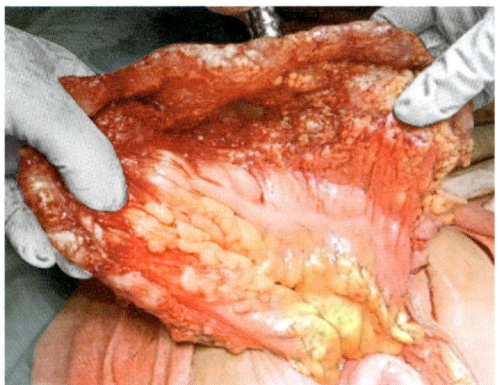

Fig. 8: Omental cake in advanced ovarian cancer.

Answer 11.1

Four other causes of upper abdominal mass are:
1. Abdominal hernia
2. Pancreatic pseudocyst
3. Abdominal lipoma
4. Cancer in stomach, liver, kidney, and colon

Answer 11.2

There is an inverse relationship between residual tumor size and survival of the patient. There is improved PFS and OS of patients who have minimal residual disease (<1 cm) at the end of surgery. Thus, optimal cytoreduction at the end of surgery is one of the most important prognostic factors of survival.

Answer 11.3

Omental cake in advanced EOC is found to be densely attached to the transverse colon. It is always possible to sharply dissect the tumor off the transverse colon without injuring the colon muscularis.

The reason behind such feasibility is as follows:
- Most of the EOCs are of serous histotype with tumor confined within the peritoneal borders of the abdominal cavity. It spreads along the peritoneal, diaphragmatic surfaces without deep invasion into abdominal organs. This allows dissection along a surgical plane between an organ and attached tumor.

Question 12

A 70-year-old lady completed treatment for advanced stage epithelial ovarian cancer with PDS and platinum-based combination chemotherapy for six cycles. She achieved complete remission. After 8 months, she developed recurrence in the form of isolated pelvic mass. The patient's ECOG (Eastern Cooperative Oncology Group) performance status was 0 and there was no ascites.

12.1. Which two modalities of treatment can be offered to the patient? (1 + 1 = 2)

12.2. Which modality of treatment is preferable? Give reasons for such preference. (1 + 1 = 2)

12.3. Outline the prognosis of the disease. (1)

Answer 12.1

The two modalities of treatment are:
1. Secondary cytoreduction followed by chemotherapy
2. Second-line chemotherapy alone

Answer 12.2

Secondary cytoreduction followed by chemotherapy.

Reasons for preference:
- Since the recurrence is isolated, the probability for complete resection is high.
- The primary tumor was platinum sensitive and disease-free interval was >6 months.

Thus, the response to platinum-based chemotherapy following secondary cytoreduction will be satisfactory.

Answer 12.3

The overall prognosis of the disease will be good with improved PFS, provided resection to no residual disease is achieved.

Question 13

A 72-year-old lady who had advanced stage epithelial ovarian tumor of mucinous subtype showed progression of disease within six months of completion of platinum-based combination chemotherapy. The patient came to the medical oncologist for help.

13.1. What is the diagnosis of disease? (1)

13.2. How should this patient be treated? (2)

13.3. Which type of treatment is suitable here? What is the prognosis of disease? (1)

Answer 13.1

Platinum-resistant ovarian cancer.

Answer 13.2

Second-line chemotherapy—single agent paclitaxel weekly or topotecan weekly or liposomal doxorubicin can be given with considerably less toxicity. These are the regimen of choice with an objective response of 10–20%.

Answer 13.3

- The treatment is palliative.
- The prognosis is very poor with OS of 9–12 months.

Question 14

A postmenopausal lady underwent PDS for advanced stage epithelial ovarian cancer. Optimum cytoreduction was achieved and the patient was referred for adjuvant chemotherapy.

14.1. Name the standard protocol of chemotherapy in this setting. (1)

14.2. Explain the benefit of maintenance therapy if added following complete response to first-line chemotherapy. (1.5)

14.3. What is the role of intraperitoneal (IP) chemotherapy in such a situation? Comment. (2.5)

Answer 14.1

Platinum-based combination chemotherapy is the standard of care in adjuvant settings.

Combination of paclitaxel and carboplatin (**Fig. 9**) is given for six cycles.

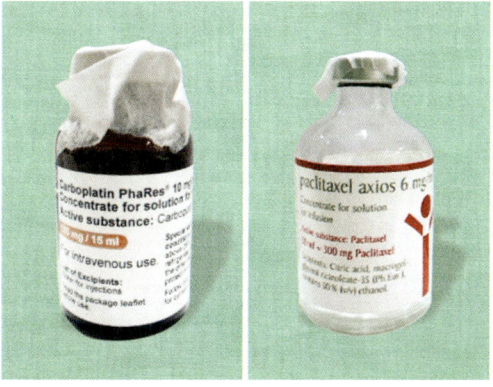

Fig. 9: Chemotherapeutic agent for ovarian cancer.

Answer 14.2

- Maintenance therapy of any of the two—paclitaxel or topotecan do not show significant difference in either PFS or OS.
- But recently poly-ADP ribose polymerase (PARP) inhibitors have shown benefit in the above two aspects.

Answer 14.3

- IP chemotherapy results in high concentration of chemotherapy with long duration of tissue exposure at the peritoneal surfaces. Thus, there is improved PFS and OS than intravenous (IV) chemotherapy. But,
- There is increased toxicity such as nausea, vomiting, pain,
- Neurotoxicity, and hematological toxicity.
- Catheter-related problems such as intestinal injury, catheter blockage, and infection is common.

Because of the above concern IP chemotherapy use is only restricted in centers that have experience to deal with the problem.

Question 15

A 67-year-old postmenopausal lady was diagnosed as advanced stage epithelial ovarian cancer. Following surgery, the histopathology revealed high-grade serous carcinoma (HGSC) **(Fig. 10)**.

15.1. Explain the origin of HGSC of ovary. (1 + 1 = 2)

15.2. How can the diagnosis of HGSC be confirmed? (1)

15.3. Justify the common stage at diagnosis of such tumor. Outline the response to chemotherapy. (1 + 1 = 2)

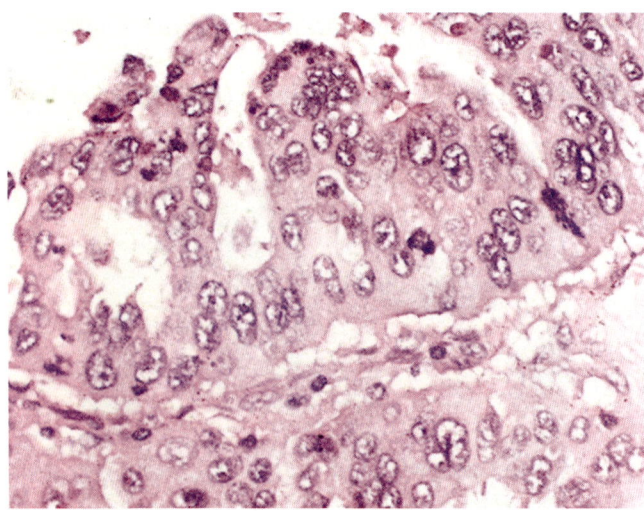

Fig. 10: High-grade serous carcinoma (HGSC) of ovary.

Answer 15.1

- HGSC mostly arises in the fallopian tube close to fimbriae from serous tubal intraperitoneal carcinoma (STIC) which is considered as the precursor of HGSC. Implantation of malignant cells from STIC to the ovary subsequently develops into a tumor mass.
- Minority of HGSC develops from peritoneal endosalpingiosis or ovarian cortical inclusion cysts.

Answer 15.2

The diagnosis of HGSC can be confirmed by a genetic mutation profile where altered genes are seen in TP53, BRCA1, and BRCA2.

Answer 15.3

- HGSC at diagnosis is most often stage III because of early dissemination by its aggressive behavior.
- The response rate to chemotherapy is high, approximately 80%.

Question 16

A 68-year-old female with advanced stage epithelial ovarian cancer is selected for neoadjuvant chemotherapy (NACT) followed by internal debulking surgery (IDS). The patient had pleural effusion **(Fig. 11)** with massive ascites.

16.1. Enumerate four unfavorable factors which favors NACT apart from those present in scenario. (0.5 × 4 = 2)

16.2. Justify the probabilities of perioperative and postoperative complications in such a case. (1 + 1 = 2)

16.3. What is the oncological outcome in this case? (0.5 × 2 = 1)

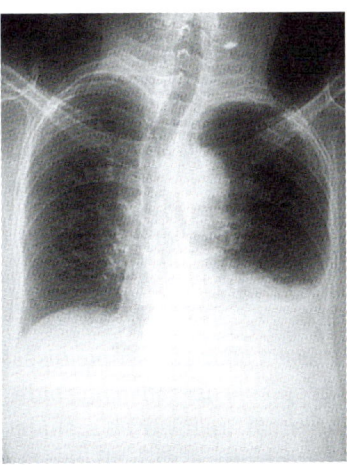

Fig. 11: Pleural effusion in left lung in ovarian malignancy.

Answer 16.1

The four unfavorable factors which favors NACT are:
1. Main tumor bulk restricted to upper abdomen.
2. Miliary spread of disease.
3. Mesenteric metastasis which would require multiple resections of the intestine.
4. Poor performance status.

Answer 16.2

The probabilities of perioperative and postoperative complications in IDS is minimum as:
- Extensive and aggressive surgery is usually not required.
- The response of NACT is good which reduces the tumor bulk and abolishes the metastases in multiple sites.

However, there might be increased blood loss due to friability of tissue which received chemotherapy (SCORPION TRIAL).

Answer 16.3

- There are no significant differences in PFS or OS between PDS and interval debulking surgery (IDS).
- The median OS and PFS is approximately 30 and 12 months, respectively.

Question 17

A 53-year-old postmenopausal lady reported with a CT scan report of complex left adnexal mass (5 × 6.8) cm with moderate ascites. There was no other metastatic evidence in CT. The patient's only complaint was the heaviness of lower abdomen for the last 15 days with early satiety.

17.1. What is the standard of care? (1)
17.2. Outline the aim of such surgery. Name the surgical procedures that are involved in this type of surgery. (1 + 2 = 3)
17.3. What is the role of chemotherapy? (1)

Answer 17.1

The standard of treatment is PDS followed by chemotherapy.

Answer 17.2

- The aim of PDS is to resect all macroscopic disease to achieve optimum cytoreduction with acceptable operative morbidity.
- The surgical procedures that are involved include:
  - Total abdominal hysterectomy with bilateral salpingo-oophorectomy

- Complete surgical staging which includes collection of ascitic fluid for cytology, abdominal exploration, omentectomy, and pelvic and para-aortic lymphadenectomy.

Answer 17.3

- Chemotherapy in advanced stage epithelial ovarian cancer is not given with curative intent. It prolongs PFS and OS of the patients following surgery.
- More than half will have complete clinical response to platinum-based regimens, with disappearance of all diseases on imaging and normalization of serum CA-125.

Question 18

A 46-year-old lady underwent cytoreductive surgery for malignant ovarian tumor. There were metastatic implants on the bowels with omental cake **(Fig. 12)**. After 24–48 hours of surgery, the patient developed abdominal distention and vomiting.

18.1. Enlist six parameters which will suggest bowel injury on immediate assessment? What investigatory findings will confirm the diagnosis.
(0.25 × 6 + 0.5 × 2 = 2.5)

18.2. Enlist three investigations in this case. (1.5)

18.3. If bowel damage happens in the transverse colon, what is the protocol of treatment? (1)

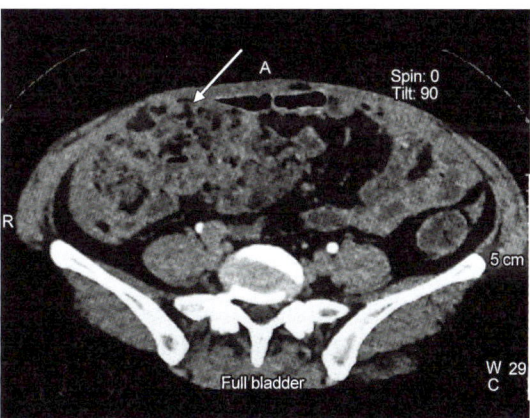

Fig. 12: Computed tomography (CT) scan showing omental cake in ovarian cancer.

Answer 18.1

1. Fever
2. Abdominal pain

3. Tenderness and guarding of abdomen
4. Dullness over frank due to free fluid
5. Tachycardia
6. Tachypnea

Findings confirming the diagnosis:
- Ultrasonography (USG) of the abdomen will show free fluid with solid particles.
- CT scan with contrast (gastrografin) of the abdomen will help to determine the site of bowel damage.

Answer 18.2

1. Blood for complete blood count (CBC)
2. Serum electrolyte
3. USG of the abdomen

Answer 18.3

- Laparotomy should be performed immediately.
- Help should be sought from surgical team who will plan the surgical procedure based on the extent of bowel injury and devitalization of tissue.

Question 19

A 43-year-old lady whose mother is suffering from HGSC attended outpatient department (OPD) for consultation. She is worried about herself and wants a thorough evaluation. After detailed history and physical examination, no abnormality was detected.

19.1. Which specific investigation should she be offered now and why? $(1 + 1 = 2)$

19.2. What preventive strategy should be adopted if the woman is found to be positive in the above investigation? $(1 \times 3 = 3)$

Answer 19.1

She should be offered genetic testing to detect breast cancer 1 (BRCA1) and BRCA2 mutations. There is 5–10% chances of having inherited predisposition to breast and ovarian cancer if BRCA1 or BRCA2 is positive. The chances are high here as her first-degree relative, i.e., the mother is suffering from HGSC.

Answer 19.2

- If the woman is BRCA positive and has completed her family, she should undergo risk reducing salpingo-oophorectomy (RRSO) bilaterally to reduce the incidence of ovarian, fallopian tube, and breast cancer.

- If the family is not yet complete, ovarian cancer screening should be continued at 6 months interval. This includes physical examination, TVS, and CA-125 until family is complete. Then RRSO should be done. The time for RRSO should not be beyond 40 years.
- In case of delay in RRSO for other than childbearing reasons, chemo prevention with oral contraception can be offered. Oral contraceptives in mutation carriers offer the same protective effect as in the general population.

Question 20

A 52-year-old postmenopausal lady underwent PDS for advanced stage epithelial ovarian cancer which was causing distress and interference in her day-to-day activities. Optimum cytoreduction **(Fig. 13)** was achieved and the patient had a smooth postoperative recovery.

20.1. How PDS alleviates symptoms and improves quality of life of the patient? (1.5 × 2 = 3)

20.2. What is the impact of optimum cytoreduction on survival? (2)

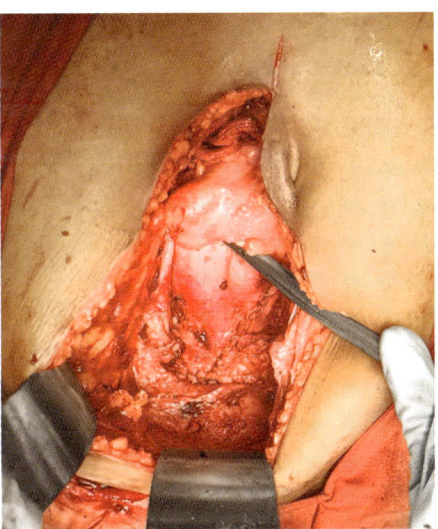

Fig. 13: Optimum cytoreduction achieved after PDS.

Answer 20.1

Primary debulking surgery removes the bulky tumor and other tumor masses, thereby alleviating symptom which presses on organs in the pelvis and upper abdomen.

Surgical removal of the tumor also reduces ascites and improves nutritional functional status of the patient, resulting in higher quality of life.

Answer 20.2

- According to evidence, there is an inverse relationship between residual tumor size and survival.
- Patients who are optimally cytoreduced had a median OS of 33.9 months versus 22.7 months for the patients who were suboptimally cytoreduced (Bristow and colleagues).

Since optimum cytoreduction was achieved in the above patient, there will be improvement in progression-free disease and OS of the patient.

Question 21

A 65-year-old female patient with advanced stage epithelial ovarian cancer was selected for NACT followed by IDS. Following surgery, the patient had incomplete response to adjuvant chemotherapy due to drug resistance.

21.1. Which chemotherapy are responsible for development of drug resistance? (1)

21.2. Which modality of treatment—PDS or IDS—diminishes the chance of drug resistance and how? (1 + 3 = 4)

Answer 21.1

Paclitaxel and carboplatin are standard first-line chemotherapy which are used in NACT or adjuvant setting in advanced staged epithelial ovarian cancer. They are responsible for causing drug resistance.

Answer 21.2

- IDS enhances the chance of drug resistance.
- PDS diminishes the chance of drug resistance by three mechanisms:
  1. PDS removes the poorly vascularized tumor, thus preventing the development of platinum resistance cancer cells in an environment of insufficient chemotherapy.
  2. In PDS when tumor is removed, there is no secretion of transcription factors, hypoxia-inducible factor 1-alpha (HIF-1α) and HIF-2α, which induce platinum resistance. Transcription factors are secreted by hypoxic cells within the bulky tumor.
  3. Platinum-resistant cancer cell clone exists in the tumor. PDS removes the tumor, thereby removing the platinum-resistant cancer cell clone.

Question 22

A 61-year-old lady presented with a hugely distended abdomen with palpable masses both in upper and lower abdomen. The patient is a poor surgical candidate and as such she was planned for NACT, but after three cycles, the response to chemotherapy was unsatisfactory.

22.1. Explain two basic reasons for unsatisfactory response to chemotherapy. (1.5 × 2 = 3)

22.2. What action should be undertaken now? (2)

Answer 22.1

The reasons for unsatisfactory response to chemotherapy includes:
- Large tumor masses have usually poor blood supply which provide a pharmacologic sanctuary where viable tumor cells escape exposure to adequate concentration of chemotherapy drugs.
- Such poorly vascularized tumor masses have large proportion of cells in the nonproliferating (G_0) phase of cell cycle, i.e., they are in low growth fraction. At this stage, they are relatively insensitive to effects of chemotherapy.

Answer 22.2

There are two options:
1. If feasible, the unfavorable factors for surgery should be corrected and IDS should be done.
2. If unfavorable factors for surgery cannot be corrected, molecular targeted agent bevacizumab can be combined with chemotherapy. There is significant improvement in PFS when bevacizumab is continued as maintenance therapy after chemotherapy.

Question 23

A 34-year-old lady presented with the history of breast cancer of her elder sister and ovarian cancer of her aunt (mother's sister). She is worried about herself and wants a thorough evaluation.

23.1. Why is the lady worried? (1)

23.2. Which specific investigation should be done in such a case? What is the probability of inheriting cancer if the investigation is positive? (1 + 1 = 2)

23.3. How the woman should be screened if genetic testing is positive? (2)

Answer 23.1

The lady is at risk for hereditary breast ovarian cancer (HBOC) syndrome which is an inherited genetic condition where breast and ovarian cancer risk is passed from generation to generation in a family.

Answer 23.2

Genetic testing should be done to detect BRCA1 or BRCA2 mutations.

There are 5–10% chances of having inherited predisposition to breast and ovarian cancer if BRCA1 or BRCA2 is positive and here the chances are higher as the disease is prevalent in the first-degree relatives (elder sister and aunt).

Answer 23.3

- Self-breast examination (SBE) monthly, beginning at the age of 18 years.
- Clinical breast examination (CBE) twice a year, beginning at the age of 25 years.
- MRI of both breasts yearly between 25 and 29 years.
- Mammogram and MRI of the breast between 30 and 50 years.
- Per vaginal (PV) examinations, TVS, and CA-125 blood test every 6-month beginning at age the 30–35 years.

Question 24

A 33-year-old lady reported with the history of breast cancer of her elder sister and ovarian cancer of her aunt (mother's sister). She is worried about herself and wants preventive measures to be taken to get rid of cancer.

24.1. If the lady has completed her family, which preventive strategy will be the best for her and why? (1 + 1 = 2)

24.2. How RRSO will prevent the development of ovarian cancer? (1 + 1 = 2)

24.3. What are the limitations of RRSO? (1)

Answer 24.1

According to National Comprehensive Cancer Network (NCCN), American College of Obstetricians and Gynecologists (ACOG), and Society of Gynecologic Oncology (SGO), RRSO will be the best for her between the ages of 35 and 40 years.

Risk reducing salpingo-oophorectomy reduces the incidence of:
- Ovarian and fallopian tube cancer by 80%
- Breast cancer by 48% particularly who are estrogen receptor (ER) positive

Answer 24.2

Risk reducing salpingo-oophorectomy will remove the fallopian tubes and ovaries on both sides. 70% of ovarian carcinomas originate from "STIC lesion" at the distal end of fallopian tube and remaining 30% originate from exfoliated tubal cells (endosalpingiosis) that implant on the ovarian surface epithelium and undergo malignant transformation. As a result, the probability of developing ovarian cancer becomes negligible.

Answer 24.3

Even after risk reducing salpingo-oophorectomy, the risk of peritoneal cancer (3.9%) persists because peritoneal malignancies can arise de novo exclusively in the peritoneum through Müllerian metaplasia.

Question 25

Carboplatin and paclitaxel combination chemotherapy is the standard of care for woman with advanced stage epithelial ovarian cancer.

25.1. What is the advantage of combining paclitaxel instead of cyclophosphamide with platinum group? (0.5 × 3 = 1.5)

25.2. Why cisplatin is replaced by carboplatin in combination chemotherapy? (0.5 × 4 = 2)

25.3. If the patient has H/O pre-existing neuropathy, which combination chemotherapy can be offered to her? (1.5)

Answer 25.1

There is significant improvement in both PFS and OS in both optimal and suboptimal debulked ovarian cancer if combination of paclitexel with platinum chemotherapy is given.

Answer 25.2

Carboplatin has less gastrointestinal tract (GIT) side effects such as nausea, vomiting as well as significantly less nephrotoxicity, neurotoxicity, and ototoxicity than cisplatin.

For this reason, carboplatin is combined with paclitaxel.

Answer 25.3

Docetaxel with carboplatin combination chemotherapy can be offered in patients with H/O pre-existing neuropathy. The efficacy of docetaxel is similar to paclitaxel but has less side effect of sensory peripheral neuropathy.

Question 26

A 44-year-old woman with advanced stage epithelial ovarian cancer with no comorbidities underwent primary cytoreduction, which was optimally debulked. She was offered adjuvant combination chemotherapy.

Epithelial Ovarian Cancer

26.1. Which combination chemotherapy among the following will be best for her and why?
- Paclitaxel and carboplatin intravenously
- Paclitaxel and cisplatin intravenously
- Docetaxel and carboplatin intravenously
- Paclitaxel and carboplatin intraperitoneally

(1 + 1 = 2)

26.2. If the patient desires to take paclitaxel and carboplatin intraperitoneally, what will be your comment? (3)

Answer 26.1

Paclitaxel and carboplatin intravenously will be best for her because evidence has shown that this results in improved PFS and OS of the patient with acceptable toxicities.

Answer 26.2

- IP chemotherapy provides a means by which high concentration of drugs and long duration of tissue exposure can be attained at the peritoneal surfaces. Thus, there is improved PFS and OS than IV chemotherapy.
- But there are concerns regarding increased toxicity—nausea, vomiting, pain, neurotoxicity, hematological toxicity, and catheter-related problems such as intestinal injury, catheter blockage, and infection.
- Because of the above concern, it is not widely used internationally. Its use is restricted only in centers that have experience to deal with IP chemotherapy.

Question 27

A 63-year-old postmenopausal lady displayed on laparotomy findings of bilateral ovarian masses with extensive dissemination of abdominal and pelvic cavities, involving the peritoneum, bowel, omentum, and other abdominal organs. The ovarian masses are multilocular, solid with extensive areas of hemorrhage and necrosis. There are friable papillae of variable sizes on the surface.

27.1. What is the likely diagnosis? Mention the tumor type according to binary system of grading. (1)
27.2. Explain your reasons for such diagnosis in relevance from the scenario. (0.5 × 4 = 2)
27.3. How can you establish the diagnosis postoperatively? (1 × 2 = 2)

Answer 27.1

The likely diagnosis is advanced stage epithelial ovarian cancer with a probability of HGSC.

Answer 27.2

High-grade serous carcinoma is the most common subtype of EOC. In the scenario:
- The patient is 63 years old.
- The tumor is aggressive with widespread dissemination.
- The tumor is bilateral.
- There are extensive areas of hemorrhage and necrosis.
- There is growth on the surface of ovaries.
- These parameters go in favor of HGSC.

Answer 27.3

The diagnosis can be established postoperatively by both immunohistochemically (IHC) and genetic mutation profile.

Immunohistochemically high-grade serous carcinoma shows:
- WT-I-+
- ER-+
- Ki-67+

Genetic mutation profile: HGSC has high mutations in P53, BRCA1, and BRCA2 oncogenes (hereditary ovarian cancer).

Question 28

A 32-year-old lady was diagnosed with advanced stage epithelial ovarian cancer at 24 weeks of gestation. The patient had H/O long-term primary infertility and is strongly desirous of continuing the pregnancy.

    28.1. What treatment plan should be preferred in such a case? (3)

    28.2. Specify the role of chemotherapy in this patient. (2)

Answer 28.1

Treatment plan of preference is as follows:
- Debulking surgery for advanced stage ovarian cancer cannot be planned when pregnancy is preferred. Thus, systemic chemotherapy should be commenced immediately and continued until fetal maturity.
- Delivery should be planned preferably by cesarean section followed by final debulking surgery.

Answer 28.2

Combination chemotherapy carboplatin and paclitaxel is the preferred regime in pregnancy.

It is given up to 35 weeks of gestation at 3 weeks' interval. There is no evidence of congenital malformation of fetus and no recordable impairment in postnatal growth, cognitive development, and cardiac function of newborn.

Question 29

A 47-year-old lady presented with a large ovarian tumor of 20 × 16 cm which is unilateral, mucinous, partly solid, and partly cystic with no evidence of dissemination elsewhere **(Fig. 14)**.

29.1. What is the probable diagnosis in the scenario? Enlist three distinguishing features that favor the diagnosis. (0.5 + 0.5 × 3 = 2)
29.2. How immunohistochemistry can help in differentiation between this tumor and metastatic mucinous carcinoma of ovary? (1.5)
29.3. Can this tumor lead to pseudomyxoma peritonei? (1.5)

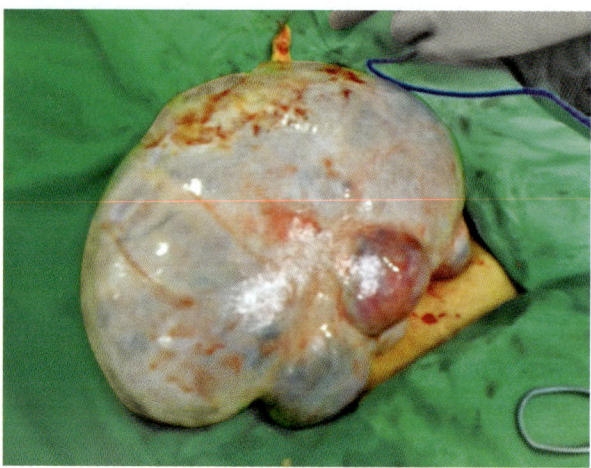

Fig. 14: Mucinous ovarian cancer.

Answer 29.1

- Primary ovarian mucinous carcinoma
- Distinguishing features in scenario are:
    1. Unilateral mass
    2. Larger than 10 cm in size
    3. Mucinous in character

Answer 29.2

Primary ovarian mucinous carcinoma is:
- CK7 is strongly positive.
- CK20 and CDX2 are relatively positive.

Metastatic mucinous carcinoma is:
- CK7 is negative.
- CK20 is positive.

Answer 29.3

Pseudomyxoma peritonei is characterized by disseminated IP mucinous tumor and mucinous ascites in the abdomen and pelvis **(Fig. 15)**. It normally starts as a slowly growing tumor from appendix and rarely from ovary. Thus, it is unlikely for this tumor to cause pseudomyxoma peritonei.

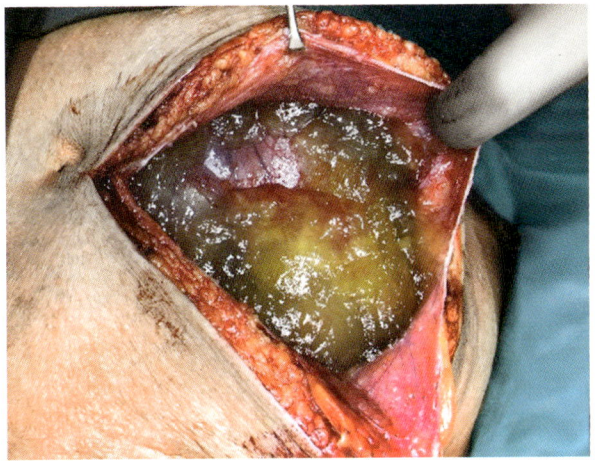

Fig. 15: Pseudomyxoma peritonei.

Question 30

A 47-year-old lady reported a bilateral ovarian tumor in CT scan. The tumors were 6 × 8 cm on the right side and 8 × 10 cm on the left side. There was evidence of extraovarian disease. On laparotomy, ovarian surface involvement was found and it was assumed to contain mucinous material.

30.1. What is the probable diagnosis? Give four reasons for the diagnosis. (1 + 0.25 × 4 = 2)

30.2. Specify confirmatory criteria on histopathology for diagnosis? (1)

30.3. What are the sites of primary tumors? (0.5 × 4 = 2)

Answer 30.1

The probable diagnosis is Krukenberg tumor or metastatic ovarian cancer **(Fig. 16)** because:
1. Tumors are bilateral (>50% of metastatic OC are bilateral).
2. Size is <10 cm.

3. Tumors are mucinous in type.
4. There is ovarian surface involvement.

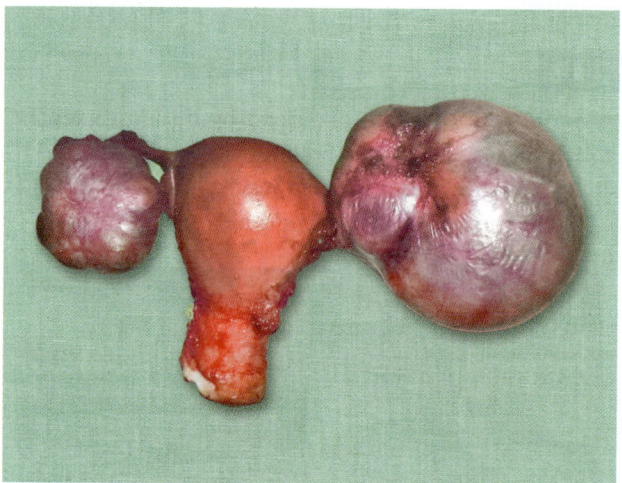

Fig. 16: Krukenberg tumor.

Answer 30.2

Histopathology will reveal mucin-filled signet ring cells in the ovarian stroma.

Answer 30.3

The five common sites of primary tumor are the colorectal, stomach, gallbladder, pancreas, and breast.

CHAPTER 7

Adnexal Mass, Germ Cell, and Sex Cord Ovarian Tumor

Question 1

A 44-year-old lady came to outpatient department (OPD) with the complaint of heaviness in the lower abdomen. Her previous ultrasonography (USG) showed adnexal mass 7 × 8 cm. She now wants evaluation.

1.1. Which imaging provides accurate characterization of adnexal mass? (0.5)
1.2. When is computed tomography (CT) scan indicated in adnexal mass? Enumerate three uses of CT scan. (1 + 0.5 × 3 = 2.5)
1.3. Enlist four characteristics in CT scan that are consistent with malignancy. (0.5 × 4 = 2)

Answer 1.1

Computed tomography scan can provide an accurate characterization of adnexal mass.

Answer 1.2

Computed tomography scan is indicated when adnexal mass is suspicious for malignancy on ultrasound.

Three uses of CT scan in adnexal mass are:
1. Characterization of adnexal mass
2. Preoperative staging
3. Determination of disease resectability

Answer 1.3

Four characteristics of CT scan **(Fig. 1)** that are consistent with malignancy are:
1. Bilateral ovarian mass
2. Cystic and solid components
3. Thick (>3 mm) irregular septa within cystic lesion
4. Papillary projections

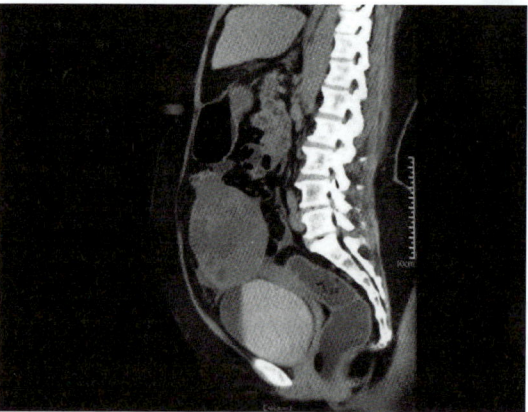

Fig. 1: Computed tomography (CT) scan showing adnexal mass.

Question 2

A 47-year-old lady presented with an adnexal mass of 9 × 6 cm in diameter. On transvaginal sonographic assessment, it revealed indeterminate findings.

2.1. Which imaging will be helpful for further assessment? How will it be helpful? (1 + 1.5 = 2.5)

2.2. If the adnexal mass is complex and shows high-signal intensity in both T1- and T2-weighted images with signal loss on fat suppression sequence, what will be the action plan? (2.5)

Answer 2.1

Magnetic resonance imaging (MRI) will be helpful because:
- It can better delineate blood, blood clots, fats, and proteinaceous materials than USG.
- It can better evaluate solid and cystic appearance through T2 signal.

Answer 2.2

- Repeat imaging and serum CA-125 after 4–6 weeks:
  - If adnexal mass is persistent or size and tumor marker increases, surgical intervention should be done.
  - The standard of care is total abdominal hysterectomy with bilateral salpingo-oophorectomy.

Question 3

A 40-year-old lady having one child after 10 years of infertility reported to the hospital with ovarian cancer. She had a definite pelvic mass 8 × 6 cm in size with ascites.

3.1. What are the risk factors in the scenario which suggest ovarian cancer? (0.5 × 2 = 1)
3.2. How do the risk factors contribute to the development of ovarian cancer? (2)
3.3. Enlist four important investigations that is helpful for diagnosis. (0.5 × 4 = 2)

Answer 3.1

- History of infertility
- Low parity

Answer 3.2

- Both infertility and low parity cause repeated ovulation which releases follicular fluid rich in inflammatory cytokines.
- Both inflammation and genetic stress cause DNA damage in the secretory epithelium of the fallopian tube.
- TP53 mutations are more likely to occur in the fallopian tube after repeated ovulation, which initiates the process of carcinogenesis.

Answer 3.3

1. Transvaginal USG with color Doppler
2. *Tumor markers:* CA-125, CA 19-9, and Cancer embryonic antigen (CEA)
3. Chest X-ray
4. CT/MRI of the whole abdomen

Question 4

A 28-year-old lady had stage I ovarian cancer at diagnosis. The frozen section at laparotomy revealed dysgerminoma.

4.1. What will be the treatment option if the patient wants to preserve fertility? (1)
4.2. Justify the performance of complete para-aortic and or pelvic lymphadenectomy in this situation. (2)
4.3. If comprehensive surgical staging is omitted at laparotomy, what will be the subsequent action? (2)

Answer 4.1

The treatment option is surgery and the preferred surgery is unilateral salpingo-oophorectomy with comprehensive surgical staging.

Answer 4.2

- There is no evidence that complete para-aortic and/or pelvic lymphadenectomy is advantageous.
- The recommendation is:
  - To palpate, the lymph nodes (LNs) and suspicious LN should be removed.
  - If no suspicious LN is detected, LN from these area should be sampled.

Answer 4.3

If comprehensive surgical staging is omitted at laparotomy, re-operation for completion of surgical staging is not needed.

The patient can be kept either on:
- Surveillance by regular pelvic and abdominal CT/MRI
- Adjuvant chemotherapy

Question 5

Dysgerminomas occurring in phenotypic females with abnormal gonads. Write a short note. (5)

Answer 5

Approximately 5% of dysgerminomas occur in phenotypic females with abnormal gonads.

Abnormal gonads may be either one of the following:
- Pure gonadal dysgenesis (46XY) or streak gonads (bilateral).
- Mixed gonadal dysgenesis (45X/46XY), unilateral streak gonads, and contralateral testis.
- Androgen insensitivity syndrome (46XY, testicular feminization).
- Thus, when the likely diagnosis is dysgerminoma in a premenarcheal patient with a pelvic mass, karyotype should be determined.

Dysgerminoma may also arise in a gonadoblastoma with gonadal dysgenesis. Though gonadoblastoma is benign ovarian tumor composed of germ cells and sex cord stroma, if left in situ with gonadal dysgenesis, >50% will sequentially develop ovarian malignancy.

In patients whose karyotype contains a Y chromosome, bilateral salpingo-oophorectomy should be done in order to avoid the risk of subsequent development of ovarian malignancy.

Question 6

Compare germ cell tumors with epithelial ovarian cancer (EOC). (5)

Answer 6

- Germ cell tumors are mostly seen between first and third decade of life, while EOCs are predominantly seen between fifth and seventh decade of life.
- Germ cell malignancies grow rapidly while epithelial ovarian tumors are slowly growing tumors.
- Abdominal distention and ascites are hallmark evidence of EOC but these symptoms are rarely seen in germ cell malignancies.
- Malignant germ cell tumors have greater predilection than epithelial tumors to metastasize hematogenously to parenchyma of liver or lung.
- Granulose cell tumor (GCT) is more commonly metastasize to LNs than EOC.
- Stage at diagnosis is mostly stage I for GCT but it is stage III for EOC.

Question 7

A 22-year-old girl presented with a rapidly growing ovarian tumor with pelvic pain. The patient came for thorough evaluation.

7.1. Based on the presentation, what is the provisional diagnosis? (1)
7.2. Outline the reason for the complaint of pelvic pain. (0.5 × 2 = 1)
7.3. After physical examination, specify the process of subsequent evaluation. (0.25 × 4 + 1 × 2 = 3)

Answer 7.1

The provisional diagnosis is germ cell tumor.

Answer 7.2

The pelvic pain is related to capsular distension, hemorrhage, or necrosis.

Answer 7.3

The subsequent process of evaluation includes laboratory tests and imaging studies.

The laboratory tests are:
- Serum alpha-fetoprotein (AFP)
- Serum human chorionic gonadotropin (hCG)
- Serum lactate dehydrogenase (LDH)
- Serum CA-125

The imaging studies are:
- Chest X-ray to exclude metastasis in lungs

- CT scan/MRI of the abdomen to document the presence and extent of retroperitoneal lymphadenopathy, liver metastasis, or metastasis in other organs.

Question 8

A 16-year-old girl presented with a unilateral solid tumor of 12 × 10 cm in size **(Fig. 2)**. Decision for unilateral salpingo-oophorectomy was taken. Postoperatively, the histopathology revealed immature teratoma, grade I.

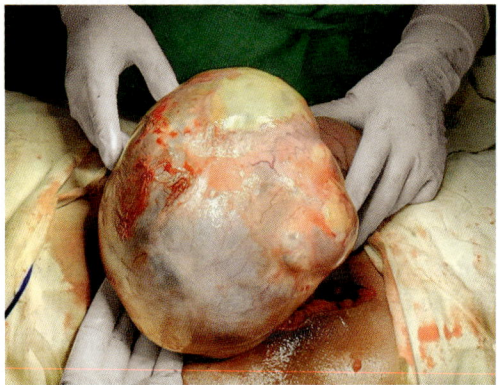

Fig. 2: Immature teratoma.

8.1. Justify whether the surgery was appropriate for the girl or not. Why the nomenclature of the tumor is immature teratoma? (1 + 0.5 = 1.5)

8.2. The patient was kept under close surveillance and she conceived twice with the outcome of two healthy children. 10 years after surgery, the patient had a relapse during surveillance. What treatment should be advised? (2)

8.3. If the disease is associated with gliomatosis peritonei, what is the prognosis? (1.5)

Answer 8.1

- Yes, the surgery was appropriate because the tumor was in stage IA, grade I and the patient was a young girl of 16 years of age.
- As the tumor contains immature neural tissue, the nomenclature is immature teratoma.

Answer 8.2

- The relapse is mostly resectable in majority cases. Thus, the treatment should be surgery with the resection of relapse organ followed by chemotherapy.

- The preferred regimen of chemotherapy is three to four cycles of BEP (bleomycin, etoposide, and cisplatin)
- Conservative approach in resection for recurrence is acceptable considering the young age of the patient and will not compromise the chances of cure because the tumors are highly sensitive to chemotherapy.

Answer 8.3

Gliomatosis peritonei means the presence of mature glial implants on peritoneal surfaces. They are not tumor derived but are teratoma-induced metaplasia and behave typically in a benign manner. Thus, the prognosis is good.

Question 9

A 24-year-old unmarried girl reported with an ultrasonographic findings of solid and cystic pelvic mass of 10 × 12 cm. 2 years before this presentation, she had undergone left oophorectomy for mature teratoma. Laboratory tests reveal:
- Serum AFP = 20,964 ng/mL
- Serum hCG = 4 IU/mL
- Serum CA-125 = 40 u/mL

9.1. What is the diagnosis? (0.5)

9.2. The laparotomy findings revealed absent left ovary, mass in the right ovary but a portion of it looked apparently healthy. Right fallopian tube and uterus were normal. Outline the standard modality of surgery that should be done. (0.5 × 3 = 1.5)

9.3. Postoperatively, which adjuvant treatment should be given? How should the patient be followed up? (1 + 2 = 3)

Answer 9.1

The probable diagnosis is yolk sac tumor (**Fig. 3**).

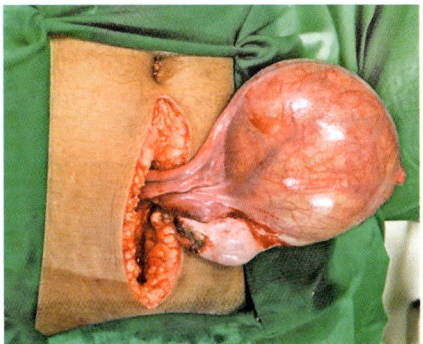

Fig. 3: Yolk sac tumor.

Answer 9.2

Considering the patient's age, desire for future childbearing, and surgical history, fertility sparing surgery should be chosen.

The operative plan should include:
- Tumor reduction by dissecting the mass away from apparently normal ovarian tissue
- Collection of 1 × 2 cm tissue from healthy part of ovary for cryopreservation
- Remodeling of remaining vascularized ovarian tissue

Answer 9.3

- Three to four cycles of BEP should be given as adjuvant treatment.
- The patient surveillance should include:
  - Serum AFP and USG at monthly and 2 monthly intervals for the first 2 years.
  - Abdominopelvic CT/MRI scan at 6 months interval
  - Thereafter the follow-up interval should be increased depending on the clinical condition.

Question 10

A 28-year-old lady reported with an advanced stage ovarian tumor with dissemination within the abdominal cavity but the other ovary was healthy. Preoperative evaluation revealed tumor markers AFP, hCG, and serum CA-125 within normal range but LDH was high. The patient is desirous of fertility sparing treatment.

10.1. Justify the feasibility and discuss the fertility sparing treatment in this case. (2)

10.2. What is the basis of fertility sparing treatment in this case? (1)

10.3. What is the late effect of BEP therapy? (1)

Answer 10.1

The probable diagnosis is advanced stage of dysgerminoma.
- Fertility sparing treatment in the form of unilateral salpingo-oophorectomy and surgical staging can be done even in the advanced stage provided the contralateral ovary is healthy.
- Surgery is followed by adjuvant chemotherapy which is BEP regimen for three to four cycles.

Answer 10.2

- The decision for fertility sparing treatment even in advanced stage is possible because of extreme sensitivity of dysgerminoma to platinum-based chemotherapy.

- The response rate to chemotherapy is excellent and patients are found without any residual lesion for a long time after completion of chemotherapy.
- Evidence has shown that there is no impact of such treatment on menstruation, reproductive function including future fertility, and overall prognosis.

Answer 10.3

Etoposide in BEP therapy is toxic and is responsible for development of secondary leukemia in the form of acute myeloid leukemia (AML) which is dose related. AML develops within 2–3 years after completion of chemotherapy.

Question 11

A 34-year-old woman with one child presented with a palpable adnexal mass which is partly solid and partly cystic. The patient had a history of menstrual irregularity, but there were no other gross abdominal findings. In preoperative evaluation, inhibin-B was 248 pg/mL in the second half of the menstrual cycle.

11.1. What is the probable diagnosis? Which histologic finding is characteristic of this diagnosis? (1 + 1 = 2)

11.2. If the disease is in stage IA, what is the stepwise approach of treatment? (2)

11.3. Enumerate the prognosis of the disease. (1)

Answer 11.1

- The probable diagnosis is granulosa cell tumor of the ovary (GCT).
- The characteristic Call–Exner bodies **(Fig. 4)** are histologically suggestive of GCT of ovary.

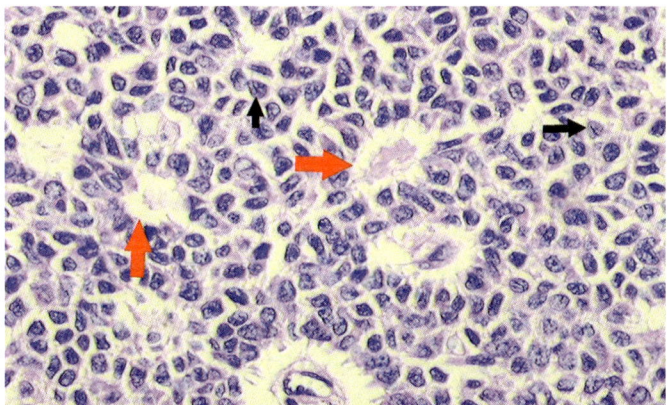

Fig. 4: Characteristic feature of Call–Exner bodies in granulosa cell tumor of ovary.

Answer 11.2

Stepwise approach of treatment:
- Dilatation and curettage to exclude coexistent adenocarcinoma of endometrium. This is followed by:
  - Unilateral salpingo-oophorectomy with limited surgical staging

Answer 11.3

Since GCT is of low-grade malignancy with indolent behavior and tumor is confined in one ovary at diagnosis, the prognosis is good with a cure rate between 70 and 90%.

Question 12

A 28-year-old girl developed unilateral ovarian mass about 10 × 12 cm size with no evidence of metastasis in the abdomen. The tumor markers were as follows:
- Serum AFP = 1,457 ng/mL
- Serum hCG = 35 IU/mL
- Serum CA-125 = 10 U/mL

12.1. What is the probable diagnosis? Which features are suggestive of the diagnosis? (1 + 1 = 2)

12.2. What is the standard conservative surgical treatment? (1.5)

12.3. Explain the role of chemotherapy in this case. Outline the prognosis of the disease. (0.5 + 1 = 1.5)

Answer 12.1

The probable diagnosis is immature teratoma.

The feature suggestive of above diagnosis are:
- *Age:* 18 years
- Unilateral ovarian tumor
- Blood tumor marker AFP and hCG are raised.

Answer 12.2

The standard conservative approach is unilateral salpingo-oophorectomy and surgical staging.

In this scenario, since the disease is in the early stage confined to one ovary and grade is I or II on frozen section, cystectomy can be done which will preserve fertility as much as possible without adversely impacting on disease-free survival and overall survival (OS). This can only be done if the tumor has developed on one pole of the ovary and the remaining ovary is healthy.

Answer 12.3

Chemotherapy in the form of BEP is only indicated if the tumor on histology reveals grade III disease. Otherwise, chemotherapy will be reserved for recurrence.

In grades I and II in this scenario, the prognosis will be excellent but it is grade III, it indicates that large quantity of immature neural tissue is present which predicts extraovarian spread and thus has poor OS.

Question 13

A 27-year-old lady, having three children presented with a recurrent pelvic mas 8 × 3.5 cm in right adnexal region 2½ years after her last child birth. She had H/O right salpingo-oophorectomy during her last cesarean section, the histology of which was GCT. The patient was on follow-up during this 2½ years' time.

13.1. What should be the treatment approach in this patient? (1.5)
13.2. During laparotomy, there was recurrent pelvic mass in right adnexa with extension into pouch of Douglas and two moderate size metastatic nodules in the omentum. Frozen section revealed recurrent granulosa cell tumor. Complete resection was done. What is the role of adjuvant chemotherapy here? (2.5)
13.3. Which tumor markers will be useful in follow-up? (1)

Answer 13.1

There is no standard approach to the management of recurrent granulosa cell tumor. Since the disease is localized, surgery will be effective.

The surgery should include cytoreduction with resection of all metastatic lesion in order to achieve complete resection leaving no residual lesion **(Figs. 5A and B)**.

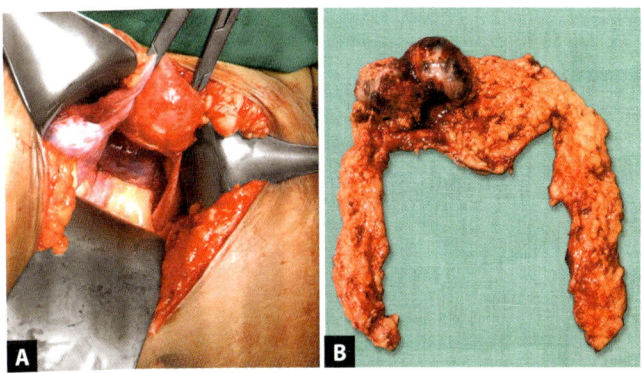

Figs. 5A and B: (A) Recurrent granulose cell tumor (GCT) in pouch of Douglas (POD); (B) Metastatic nodule in omentum.

Answer 13.2

The role of chemotherapy following complete resection of recurrent granulosa cell tumor is controversial.

- Studies have shown adjuvant chemotherapy after secondary cytoreduction with no residual tumor did not prolong the progression-free survival (PFS) or OS of the patient. Thus, the authors recommended to omit chemotherapy in patients who have no residual disease after surgery.
- But recent studies have suggested that adjuvant chemotherapy improves the therapeutic outcome and prognosis in regards to the occurrence of second relapse. National Comprehensive Cancer Network (NCCN) guidelines recommend therefore to use postoperative chemotherapy for women with completely resected disease in both advanced stage and recurrent disease.

Acceptable chemotherapy options include BEP, EP, PAC and carboplatin and paclitaxel. Carboplatin and paclitaxel are commonly used now-a-days in view of their better tolerance.

Answer 13.3

Inhibin B and anti-Müllerian hormone (AMH) are useful tumor markers in follow-up of patient.